WARD

FAMILY HEAL

C000071484

LIVING V
HEART CONDITION

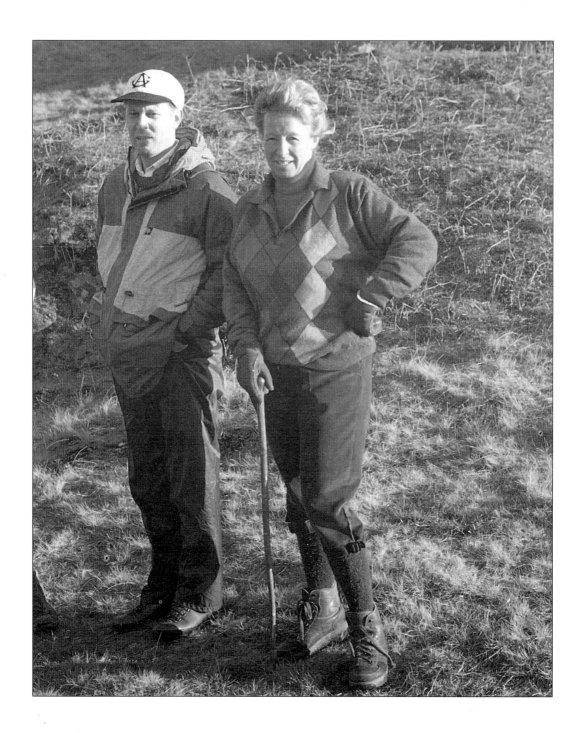

WARD LOCK

FAMILY HEALTH GUIDE

LIVING WITH A
HEART CONDITION

DR MICHAEL TURNER AND ANGELA DICKINSON

IN ASSOCIATION WITH
THE FAMILY HEART ASSOCIATION

WARD LOCK

Dr Michael Turner and Angela Dickinson

Dr Michael Turner, a life scientist, has worked for the National Health Service and the Medical Research Council and spent 12 years in the University of Southampton. He was formerly Director General of the British Nutrition Foundation and is currently Chief Executive of the Family Heart Association. Angela Dickinson has a background in specialist nursing and nutrition, working mainly in hospitals in Oxford.

A WARD LOCK BOOK

First published in the UK 1995
by Ward Lock
Wellington House
125 Strand
London
WC2R 0BB

A Cassell Imprint
Copyright © Text Dr Michael Turner 1995

Illustrations Ward Lock 1995

Distributed in the United States
by Sterling Publishing Co., Inc.
387 Park Avenue South, New York, NY 10016-8810

Distributed in Australia
by Capricorn Link (Australia) Pty Ltd
2/13 Carrington Road, Castle Hill, NSW 2154

A British Library Cataloguing in Publication Data block for this book may be obtained from the British Library

ISBN 0 7063 7405 3
Designed by Lindsey Johns and typeset by The Design Revolution, Brighton
Printed and bound in Spain

Acknowledgements

The authors are most grateful to Professor Tony Winder of the Royal Free Hospital, London, and Dr Richard Wray of the Conquest Hospital, Hastings, for checking the accuracy of the medical and scientific content of the book and for general comment on the text; and to Miss Sarah Woodman for her administrative support. We also thank Helen Denholm, commissioning editor, of Ward Lock and Ruth Baldwin, who edited the manuscript, for their contribution.
Acknowledgements are also due to the following for providing photographs:
Camera Talks (Pages 36, 37, 38 and 39); Family Heart Association (Pages 18 and 19); National Dairy Council (Pages 61, 63, 64, 67 and 68); Life File (remaining photographs).
Cover photograph: Comstock Picture Library.

Contents

Introduction

As we get older, the body wears out. Sooner or later, one of the body's vital systems fails and we die. Often it is the heart or circulation that fails first.

When angina and heart attack occur in old age it should not, therefore, be a matter for surprise: after all, we have to die of something. But when they occur in younger people, these problems are a reason for major public health concern.

Heart attack is the most common cause of death in the UK as in most developed countries throughout the world and, with angina, is a frequent cause of disability. It seems that life in developed countries favours premature degeneration of the arteries, especially the coronary arteries that carry blood to the heart.

The irony is that angina and heart attack can be delayed, or even avoided altogether, by prudent eating and living. There is no need to die or be disabled by these diseases while young. In countries where low-fat living is the norm, coronary heart disease is rare, as it was rare in the UK during the low-fat war years between 1939 and 1945. Prudence need not be boring, and surely it is better to have more fun-filled active years than be disabled or dead from premature angina or heart attack.

This book gives the facts about angina and heart attack, and explains how to delay or avoid them. But if you or a member of your family are unfortunate enough to suffer these problems already, the book also tells you what might happen in hospital, what treatments you might expect and how to order your eating and living to reduce the chance of angina getting worse or of having a second heart attack in the near future.

Michael Turner
Angela Dickinson

Chapter one

How does the heart circulate blood?

The circulation

Every tissue in the body needs oxygen, calories and nutrients for growth and repair, and to do their job, whatever that might be.

All of the tissues – muscle, brain, liver, for example, even bones and teeth – do chemical work. Some are more chemically active than others and need more fuel (calories) and more oxygen to 'burn' the fuel. Thus the brain needs more than bone, the liver more than skin. In addition to chemical work, muscle also does physical work, so needs extra fuel and oxygen.

The oxygen, calories and nutrients needed by the tissues are carried in the blood which is transported to the tissues in the arteries, thick-walled muscular yet flexible tubes. The arteries divide into a network of very thin blood vessels, the capillaries, which reach every part of the tissue to exchange oxygen and nutrients for carbon dioxide and other waste chemicals. Capillaries are so small that a microscope is needed to see them.

The stale blood that has given up oxygen, calories and nutrients, and which has picked up waste materials, is carried away in the veins which are less muscular than the arteries. The blood vessels that stand out on the back of the hands are veins. The pulse in your wrist is an artery.

The stale blood is returned to the heart, then passed through the lungs to replenish the oxygen. Calories and nutrients are added from the liver and other body stores. Waste materials are disposed of by the liver, kidneys and intestines.

The heart

To get blood around the body a pump is needed; the heart does that job. When you feel your pulse, you are feeling the surge of blood in an artery when the heart beats. The pulse should be strong and regular, though it is entirely normal for it to speed up a bit when you breathe in and slow down again as you breathe out. It also speeds up when you take exercise, to provide more blood to the muscle.

The most active of all the tissues is the heart which, in an 80-year lifespan, beats more than 3,000 million times. It is especially important

7

How does the heart circulate blood?

therefore for the heart muscle itself to be well nourished, to have its own blood supply.

Heart muscle is supplied by a network of arteries, the coronary arteries, which divide, as elsewhere, into smaller blood vessels and finally into the very fine capillaries. If the coronary arteries become blocked, the heart muscle will be starved of oxygen. When that happens, there is pain. Some damage to the heart muscle itself can occur. Eventually there may be a heart attack, which could result in death. Sometimes, however, the heart is able to adapt to small blockages by finding a new route for the blood, thus minimizing the effect of the blockage.

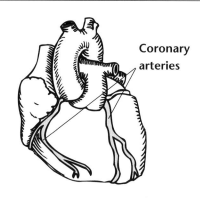

Coronary arteries

The coronary arteries supply the heart itself with oxygen, calories and nutrients. When the coronary arteries become partially or totally blocked, angina, heart attack or death result.

How the heart works

The heart is really two pumps in one. The right-hand side of the heart receives stale blood that has already been round the body, and pumps it to the lungs to get rid of waste carbon dioxide and pick up oxygen. The fresh oxygenated blood is returned to the left-hand side of the heart, which then pumps it round the rest of the body. The coronary arteries which supply the heart itself branch off from the aorta, the main artery coming out of the heart. The heart, therefore, gets the best fresh blood, richest in life-giving oxygen.

The heart has two compartments on each side, four in all. The right atrium (sometimes called the right auricle) receives the stale blood that has already been round the body. The right atrium is separated from the right ventricle by a valve. Blood is pumped from the right atrium into the right ventricle which then pumps the stale blood up to the lungs to expel waste carbon dioxide and pick up fresh oxygen.

Freshly oxygenated blood is returned from the lungs to the left atrium which is separated from the left ventricle by a valve. Blood is pumped from the left ventricle through the aortic valve into the aorta, the main blood vessel which supplies, through its many branches, the entire body. The main coronary arteries are the first branches off the aorta.

This book concentrates on angina and heart attack. Other heart disorders, such as valve problems, hole-in-the-heart conditions and heart pacemaker malfunction, are not dealt with here.

For more information about these other problems contact the British Heart Foundation which specializes in information on surgical treatments for heart conditions (see page 79 for the address).

Chapter two

What is angina and heart attack?

Angina

Angina means pain in the heart. When the blood supply to the heart muscle is inadequate, pain in the chest will usually occur, and this may spread to the neck, arms and shoulders. The pain may be accompanied by breathlessness or a feeling of suffocation, especially on exertion – going upstairs or running for a bus, for example. In severe cases, angina symptoms may occur even while sitting or standing. Sometimes people have mild angina for many years without seeking medical advice, especially if breathlessness is not a feature and the pain is not severe.

Plaque, the cause of angina

Angina is caused by partial blockage of the coronary arteries with fatty and fibrous deposits in the artery wall. The lining of the arteries grows lumpy and rough, instead of smooth, and the arteries become stiff because of fibrous deposits rather than flexible (this is known as hardening of the arteries). The width of the coronary arteries is reduced as the fatty fibrous lumps, called plaque, get bigger.

Even when the width of the coronary arteries is reduced substantially and cannot stretch properly to carry extra blood during exercise – because they are more rigid than they should be (hardened) – enough blood may still get through to support a sedentary lifestyle, although there may be discomfort on unfamiliar exertion. But if the coronary arteries become more blocked than that, chest pain with or without breathlessness will be felt – and should be acknowledged as a warning that some sort of remedial action is urgently needed. The body uses pain to indicate danger. Take particular note of chest pain: it may only be indigestion, but could be an early warning that a heart attack is imminent.

A lot can be done to help angina sufferers and to prevent angina leading on to a heart attack. The earlier action is taken, the better. Go and see your doctor.

It may only be a question of making corrective adjustments to eating and living habits, with drugs in reserve in case of crisis. Or it may be necessary to go on drugs, diet and lifestyle therapy for life. In severe cases surgery may be required. It all depends on the nature and severity of the medical problem.

Whatever treatments you have, most people find it helpful to understand the nature of the problem and the reason for the treatment.

What is angina and heart attack?

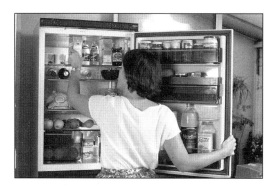

It may be necessary for angina sufferers to make corrective adjustments to eating and living habits.

How plaque is formed

With blood rushing round the arteries and veins under pressure, it is inevitable that there should be wear and tear, small damage to the lining of the blood vessels. This is most evident in the arteries near the heart, the aorta and the coronary arteries, which feed the heart itself. These small lesions are entirely normal and are repaired just as a small surface cut or graze to the skin is repaired. A small clot forms and the tissue is rebuilt.

Sometimes, however, the small 'initial lesion' does not repair normally, especially with repeated injury at the same site. Cholesterol and other fats penetrate the inner lining of the artery. Some research suggests that this is more likely when the fats in the blood are chemically damaged, and form oxidized fat, and that antioxidant vitamins (carotene, vitamin C and vitamin E) and antioxidant minerals (notably selenium) may help by slowing down the oxidation of fats, but this is by no means certain.

The invasion of the inner lining of the arteries by cholesterol and other fats provokes one of the body's defence reactions. Scavenger cells (macrophages) in the blood follow the oxidized fat into the arterial wall and ingest the fat. That is how the body deals with invading organisms or foreign chemicals. Macrophages that become bloated with fat are then called foam cells. As more and more cholesterol and other fats invade the wall of the artery, a fat-filled lump is formed. Meanwhile the lump is wrapped up in fibre, another of the body's defences. The result is plaque – a fatty lump

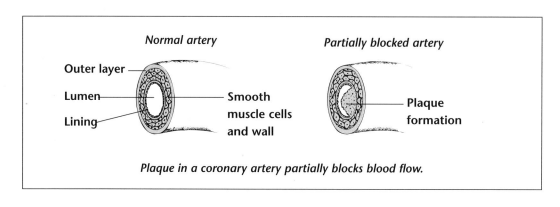

Plaque in a coronary artery partially blocks blood flow.

with a fibrous cap and possibly a fibrous mesh running through it which, in fact, is helpful in giving the plaque greater stability. It is unstable plaque without a fibrous mesh that causes problems.

In most cases, plaque forms equally all round the artery and is then called concentric plaque. When that happens, the effect is similar to the furring-up of a water pipe. Sometimes the plaque may be on one side only, and it is then known as eccentric plaque. Eccentric plaque is more likely to burst and is therefore more dangerous.

When the fibrous cap covering plaque splits, the plaque bursts, the body perceives this as tissue injury and a massive clot forms to plug the gap. This is the classic 'coronary thrombosis'. The clot can block blood flow totally, causing a heart attack. Sometimes a clot forms without rupture of the plaque, just because the lining of the artery is rough rather than smooth as it should be. This is made more likely if the clotting tendency of the blood is increased.

Heart attack

When a blood clot forms in a coronary artery already narrowed by plaque, the blood supply to the heart muscle can be cut off completely. When that happens the heart muscle is starved of oxygen and dies. Depending where the blockage occurs – in short, how much heart muscle is deprived of life-giving oxygen – one of two things occurs. Either part of the heart is damaged but the heart continues beating, or the heart is so seriously damaged that it stops altogether and death results.

When a heart attack takes place, the task facing the doctors and other health professionals is to keep the heart going long enough for the blockage, the clot, to be dissolved and blood flow to the heart muscle restored. Speed is essential. Many patients who die of a heart attack do so during the first two hours of the attack. That is why calling an ambulance without delay is so important. Even before paramedics or a doctor arrive on the scene there are things family, friends or passers-by can do to help. Emergency resuscitation techniques are described later in this book (see pages 43–7).

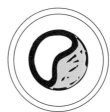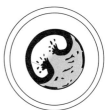

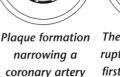

Plaque formation narrowing a coronary artery   *The cap over plaque rupturing – often the first event in a heart attack*

When the fibrous cap covering plaque ruptures, massive clotting and heart attack occur. The task is to 'stabilize' existing plaque to reduce the risk of it rupturing.

Chapter three

Causes of angina and heart attack

Blood clotting

A heart attack is usually brought on by a blood clot forming at the site of atherosclerotic plaque in a coronary artery.

It is necessary for blood to clot when tissue injury occurs. If it did not, there would be a risk of continued bleeding, perhaps even death, from a small cut or bruise. That is the problem haemophiliacs face.

On the other hand, it is not good for blood to clot excessively or when it is not necessary. That could lead to blockages in the circulation, precisely what happens in a heart attack.

The clotting process

When there is tissue injury on the outside of the body – a cut or a bruise, for example – damage occurs to the tiny blood vessels, the capillaries. The blood vessels supplying the damaged area then constrict, in an attempt to minimize blood loss. The platelets, the tiniest of the blood cells, clump together and stick to the damaged blood vessels in an attempt to stop blood leaking out. This is a temporary repair a bit like putting your finger into the hole when your garden hose bursts.

Then comes the permanent repair job. Platelets clumping together trigger a massive clotting of the blood. A soluble protein, fibrinogen, is rapidly converted to its insoluble form, fibrin, which forms a large glutinous blob which re-forms into a mesh of tough fibres at the site of the injury to hold it together and stop blood leaks. The clot progressively shrinks. As it does so, it pulls the damaged surfaces together to facilitate repair. That is the scab you get when, for example, you graze your knee. If the injury is internal, however, a scab forms inside. If the injury is to the lining of a blood vessel, as can occur in atherosclerosis, a clot and scab will form there.

In coronary arteries made rough by plaque, the blood may clot even without further tissue injury, causing a blockage. But clotting normally occurs when a plaque, the cholesterol-filled bulge in the arteries, bursts. The blood reacts to this as tissue injury and goes into its clotting routine, blocking the blood flow and damaging the heart in the process.

Clotting is more likely if fibrinogen levels are higher than normal, or if a blood enzyme involved in the clotting process, Factor VII, is excessive. The levels of both are raised by a high-fat diet, as also is the tendency for platelets to clump together when they should not.

Thrombolysis, the breaking-down of blood clots

Everything in the healthy body is in a state of balance or equilibrium. That is true of blood clotting too. In addition to the blood-clotting mechanism there is a balancing mechanism for breaking down clots. That way, if too large a clot forms, the excess is dissolved. The process of breaking down blood clots is called thrombolysis.

Just as excessive blood clotting is a hazard that might bring on a heart attack, a sub-standard clot-dissolving facility (reduced thrombolysis activity) is also a hazard.

Coronary heart disease risk factors

It is rare for angina or heart attack to have a single cause, though this can happen. Usually several 'risk factors' combine. The particular combination of risk factors can vary from individual to individual. Thus, for example, one person may have a heart attack because of diabetes, high blood pressure and drinking too much alcohol, while the cause in another patient may be high blood cholesterol, smoking and insufficient physical activity.

There are a great many risk factors for which there is some evidence of an association with coronary heart disease. Some can be modified, others cannot. There are 11 modifiable risk factors of major medical importance. The 'big three' are high blood cholesterol, high blood pressure and smoking.

Risk factors for coronary heart disease

Can be modified
- High blood cholesterol
- High blood pressure
- Smoking
- Obesity
- Diabetes
- Inactivity
- Excess alcohol intake
- High blood triglyceride (see pages 16 and 19)
- Low blood HDL (see pages 16-17)

- High blood fibrinogen
- High blood Factor VII

Unavoidable
- Getting older
- Being male
- Being post-menopausal
- Genetic disorders, including a family history of premature angina or heart attack

Causes of angina and heart attack

Blood cholesterol

It has become abundantly clear in recent years that a raised blood cholesterol is almost a pre-requisite for angina and heart attack. If cholesterol is very low, you may get away with smoking, high blood pressure and obesity; if blood cholesterol is elevated, you become sensitized to the effects of smoking and other risk factors. Getting cholesterol down, therefore, is a major public health priority.

What exactly constitutes a raised blood cholesterol? The average total blood cholesterol in Britain is 5.8 millimoles per litre (mmol/l). This cannot be used to define 'normal'; it is significantly higher than the target value of 5.2 mmol/l which is the *top* end of the healthy zone. Even 5.2 mmol/l is too high if other risk factors are present, especially in middle-aged men. By world standards 5.2 mmol/l is high.

The higher the total cholesterol, the higher the risk of death from coronary heart disease. At the upper end of the spectrum, above 7.8 mmol/l, risk escalates alarmingly. Some people have genetic defects that affect blood cholesterol. They suffer from FH (familial hypercholesterolaemia) or FCH (familial combined hyperlipidaemia). People with FH or FCH may have a total blood cholesterol of 10–20 mmol/l which is why, if not diagnosed and treated early, they generally die young in their fifties, forties or thirties – sometimes even younger than that (see 'Inherited high cholesterol' on page 17).

In Britain today less than 30 per cent of the population have a total blood cholesterol within the healthy zone of 3.5 to 5.2 mmol/l. The other 70 per cent are at increased risk of

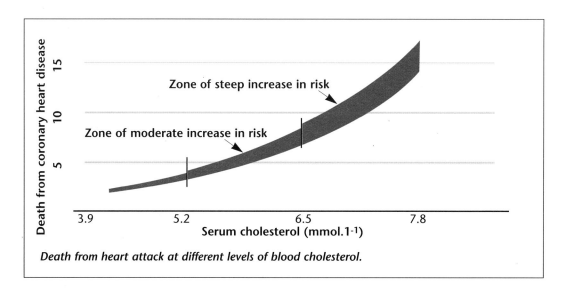

Death from heart attack at different levels of blood cholesterol.

14

angina or heart attack, and sensitized to the damaging effects of other risk factors. It is not surprising that the UK is near the top of the international league table for deaths from coronary heart disease.

Age and blood cholesterol

The young have more to gain relatively from reducing their blood cholesterol than the old, though *everyone* will benefit to some extent (see the table on page 16). A 10 per cent reduction in total blood cholesterol can be achieved by diet alone, which can reduce coronary heart disease risk by half.

Different types of blood cholesterol

Anyone with an elevated total cholesterol, certainly if above 6.5 mmol/l, should, ideally, have a more detailed analysis of the different types of cholesterol, and other fats, in the blood. They also require a full medical assessment including other risk factors such as blood pressure, smoking, family history and so on. This is a daunting task in Britain where nearly 30 per cent of the population have a blood cholesterol of 6.5 or more.

The different types of cholesterol and other fats in the blood are many and various. Fats and cholesterol circulating freely in the blood would quickly clog up the circulation and kill you. Most are, therefore, transported as tiny particles called lipoproteins, so small that they are invisible to the naked eye. In this form they mix with the watery plasma in the blood and do not clump together, so lipoproteins are a suitable way of transporting fatty substances.

Death from heart attack in the UK and other countries

(per 100,000 of the population aged 35–74 years in 1990)

	Men	Women
Czechoslovakia	609	218
Northern Ireland	566	213
Scotland	562	241
Ireland	514	171
Finland	508	154
England and Wales	448	167
New Zealand (1989)	439	162
Denmark	418	152
USA (1989)	322	132
Germany	289	92
Greece	218	69
Switzerland	214	58
Portugal	176	65
Japan	57	23

Source: CHD Statistics, BHF/CPG (1993).

All lipoproteins contain different types of fat (cholesterol, triglycerides, phospholipid) and proteins, but in varying amounts.

The risk of coronary heart disease is increased as the low-density lipoprotein (LDL) increases; it is the true villain of the piece. High-density lipoprotein (HDL), on the other hand, is protective. It mops up surplus cholesterol and returns it safely to the liver for reuse or disposal. Thus it is helpful to have a low LDL (less than 3.4 mmol/l) and a high HDL (more than 1 mmol/l).

Causes of angina and heart attack

Changes in LDL and HDL with age

Children before puberty have a higher HDL than adults. After puberty, HDL falls in boys but not in girls, which may account for the lower incidence of angina and heart attack in middle-aged women. But during and after the menopause women lose this protection and their HDL comes down to the level found in men. As a consequence, coronary heart disease rates rise in post-menopausal women.

The loss of HDL in women associated with the menopause can be prevented by hormone replacement therapy (HRT). As a bonus, HRT also prevents the bone loss that leads to osteoporosis which is especially common in older women. For these reasons there are many doctors who advocate offering HRT to all women reaching the menopause. There are slight concerns that uterus (womb) and breast cancer rates are higher in women receiving HRT, but the benefits in reducing death from coronary heart disease and disability from osteoporosis-related injury outweigh any

Lipoproteins and other fats in the blood and what they do

Low-density lipoprotein (LDL)
Carries cholesterol from the liver, where it is made, around the body to the tissues where it is used.

High-density lipoprotein (HDL)
Carries surplus cholesterol not used by the tissues back to the liver for disposal.

Triglyceride (TG)
Ordinary fat used as a 'fuel'. It is transported in lipoproteins, especially in VLDLs and chylomicrons.

Very low-density lipoprotein (VLDL)
Transports triglycerides from where they are made around the body to the tissues where they are used.

Chylomicrons
Especially rich in triglycerides. They transport dietary fat absorbed in the intestines to the liver for processing and to fat tissues for storage.

disadvantages. In any case, the nature of HRT has improved in recent years, further reducing the small risk of cancer of the womb. However, it is a matter of individual choice.

Genetic disorders

Some people, through no fault of their own, or of their parents, inherit a tendency to high cholesterol, high blood pressure or diabetes, all of which predispose them to (that is, make them more likely to have) premature coronary heart disease. But the fact that the problem is genetic does not mean that nothing can be done. It just means that you may need drugs when others might manage with diet and other lifestyle measures alone, or that you have to be more disciplined in your diet and lifestyle to cope with the situation.

Inherited high cholesterol

The two main genetic disorders causing high cholesterol are familial hypercholesterolaemia (FH) and familial combined hyperlipidaemia (FCH).

In FH, cholesterol (more specifically the LDL) cannot get out of the blood fast enough, so tends to accumulate, building to very high levels, often 10 mmol/l or more. In FCH, cholesterol is produced and secreted into the blood (as LDL) too fast, so again it tends to accumulate.

FH is a more serious condition than FCH, but both give a good chance of early angina or heart attack if not diagnosed and treated. It always comes back to this – *early* diagnosis is so important. Yet it is this aspect of public health which is most neglected. There are at present no community-based programmes in the UK to detect people with inherited high cholesterol.

An estimated 0.2 per cent of the population of the Western world carries FH gene defects and up to 1 per cent carries FCH gene defects, according to the International Atherosclerosis Society. In Britain that means 100,000 people with the FH gene and more than 500,000 with FCH. Some people regard this figure for FCH as an overestimate but, however you look at it, there are a great many people in Britain who inherit a high cholesterol and are at serious risk of angina or heart attack in their thirties, forties or fifties (sometimes in their twenties or even teens). Less than 10 per cent of people with FH or FCH have so far been identified, diagnosed and treated.

Lumps and bumps

How can you know if you have inherited high cholesterol? The only certain diagnosis requires a visit to your doctor, a blood test, medical examination and consideration of your family history of coronary heart disease and other illnesses. Present resources are insufficient for doctors to test the entire population, but there are things you can do to help you decide if you are perhaps at risk, and put yourself at the head of the queue for a full medical examination.

For a start, look at the pictures on page 18 and ask yourself if you have any of the outward signs of high cholesterol – lumps, bumps and rings. Do members of your family (blood relatives) tend to die young from heart attack or suffer from angina? If so, tell your doctor.

The important thing to remember is that, if you know you have a problem, you can deal

Causes of angina and heart attack

with it. Ignorance may be more blissful but, in this instance, gives you an 80 per cent risk of dying young if you ignore the problem. Exactly how to deal with the problem of elevated cholesterol, whether inherited or not, is described in detail in Chapter six.

Have you inherited high blood cholesterol?

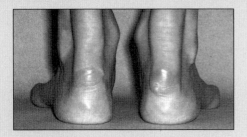

Thickening of the Achilles tendon in familial hypercholesterolaemia (xanthoma).

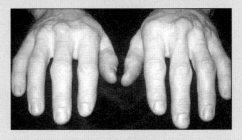

Cholesterol deposits on the knuckles in familial hypercholesterolaemia (xanthoma).

- Do people in your family tend to suffer from angina or die young from heart attack before 50 years of age (men) or 60 years of age (women)?
- Is the Achilles tendon at the back of your ankle thickened?

- Do you have mysterious knobs on your knuckles?
- Do you have yellow patches or flaps on the skin around the eyes?
- If you are under 50, do you have a white ring around the coloured part of your eye?

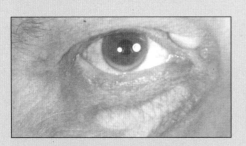

Cholesterol deposits around the eyes in familial hypercholesterolaemia (xanthelasmata).

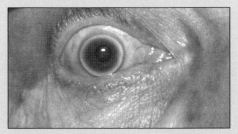

Cholesterol ring in the eye in familial hypercholesterolaemia (corneal arcus).

Blood triglycerides

Cholesterol is the number one killer if high blood levels are maintained for any length of time. But cholesterol is not the only killer fat. Raised triglyceride is also a problem; it makes blood clot when it need not, or clot excessively when a small clot might be more appropriate to repair a small injury.

Triglycerides are the same type of fats as you find on meats, in dairy produce, vegetable oils and so on. They cannot be allowed to circulate freely in the blood as fat droplets; the fat droplets would come together and clog up the smaller blood vessels, causing all sorts of problems, including heart attack. Instead triglyceride is wrapped up in tiny microscopic packages, the lipoproteins (already described on pages 15–16), just as cholesterol is. Triglycerides are found mainly in very low-density lipoproteins (VLDLs) and, after eating, in chylomicrons as well.

Triglycerides from food are absorbed in the intestines and transported initially as chylomicrons, the largest of all the lipoproteins.

These are removed from the blood by the liver and repackaged as the smaller VLDLs for distribution to the fat stores and to muscle, where they can be burned as 'fuel'.

Triglyceride is at its highest after a fatty meal and can make the plasma of the blood, which is normally clear and transparent, turn 'milky' in appearance. If blood taken after a meal is left in a bottle to settle, the fat would rise to the top as a separate fatty layer.

After a fatty meal, blood clotting is easily provoked. The health message, therefore, is not only to eat a diet which is low in fat but also to spread that fat throughout the day, to avoid surges in blood triglycerides which, for anyone with a lot of plaque or angina, could prove dangerous.

Saturated fats have a stronger clotting influence than monounsaturates or polyunsaturates, but all fats tend to trigger the clotting mechanism. There is no doubt, therefore, about the dietary message: go easy on fats, especially saturated fats.

High blood pressure

High blood pressure is quite common in developed countries, especially in older people.

To get blood round the body in the arteries and veins, it is necessary to maintain a certain head of pressure – the blood pressure.

When you have your blood pressure measured, you are given two numbers. The bigger number relates to the surge in pressure each time the heart beats and pumps blood around the body. This is called systolic blood pressure. The second number is the minimal blood pressure as the heart relaxes and refills between heart beats, and is called diastolic blood pressure. Both values, systolic and diastolic, are relevant and measure different things. Risk of coronary heart disease relates

Causes of angina and heart attack

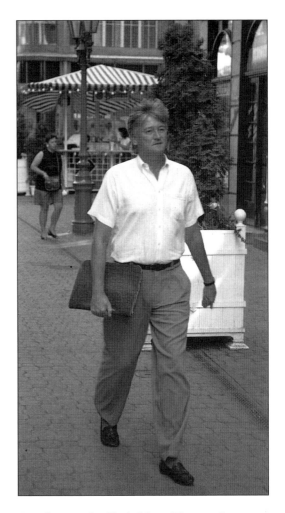

Regular exercise like brisk walking can improve heart health.

separately to both systolic and diastolic blood pressure, though in most cases, when one is elevated, so is the other.

A typical blood pressure reading might be 120/70: that is, a systolic blood pressure of 120mm of mercury or Hg (the unit used to measure it – no need to worry about units) and a diastolic pressure of 70.

In the UK, as in all developed countries, blood pressure rises with age. This does not occur in people with a simpler, more 'peasant' style of living. So we conclude that blood pressure does not need to rise with age – and it would be a good thing if it did not, because high blood pressure is associated with strokes and, to a lesser extent, with heart attacks.

What causes high blood pressure?

You are more likely to have high blood pressure if you are obese, inactive, eat a high-fat or high-salt diet and drink too much alcohol. The clue to preventing high blood pressure is to be found in the known causes: watch your weight, go easy on alcohol and salt, be active and contain stress within reasonable limits. How to do these things is explained later in this book.

Inherited high blood pressure

It is probable that some people inherit a tendency to high blood pressure, though this is less clear cut than for cholesterol. However, high blood pressure does tend to run in families. The dietary and lifestyle measures described later in this book to promote better heart health will assist also with reducing blood pressure if this is raised above an acceptable level. Of particular importance are maintaining body weight at a healthy level, containing alcohol consumption to a moderate amount and limiting salt consumption. Regular exercise (like walking, swimming, cycling and dancing) can help, as can stress reduction. There is some evidence that the soothing effect of regularly stroking a cat or dog, even a human, helps reduce excess blood pressure.

Smoking

After high blood cholesterol, smoking is perhaps the next most likely factor to precipitate a heart attack. Smoking increases both the tendency to form plaque (atherosclerosis) and the clotting of blood (thrombosis). How precisely these effects of smoking occur is not yet entirely clear. But there is no doubt that smoking kills, either from a heart attack or cancer.

Smoking in Britain has been decreasing slowly but steadily in recent years, yet still a worrying 30 per cent of the population are regular smokers. Even more worrying, smoking is on the increase among children, teenagers, and young women. More than 10 per cent of 11–15-year-olds are regular smokers. The number of smokers is higher in older schoolchildren: up to 25 per cent. (Source: ASH, 1994.)

Anyone suffering angina or heart attack is at particular risk and must stop smoking to improve their health prospects. The benefit of quitting begins immediately, but increases progressively over a period of years. Remember: coronary prevention is a lifetime commitment, a commitment for life. Giving up is difficult but can be done and must be done. For help with how to quit smoking see page 68.

Diabetes

Diabetes is the result of a number of defects in the control of body chemistry. Most noticeable is excess sugar in the blood which spills over into the urine. But there are faults also in the way the body handles proteins and fats.

Diabetes more than doubles the risk of death from coronary heart disease, which is the main cause of death in diabetics as indeed it is

Causes of angina and heart attack

in the population as a whole.

Diabetes occurs in two forms. The more severe requires treatment with daily insulin injections and affects about 100,000 people in the UK. It is called insulin-dependent diabetes (IDD). Quite simply, the body does not produce enough insulin, so extra has to be provided by the daily injections. The milder form of diabetes, which affects half a million or more in the UK, is called non-insulin-dependent diabetes (NIDD), and does not usually require insulin injections. In NIDD ample insulin is produced in the body; indeed often there is more than in non-diabetics. But the tissues of the body do not respond properly to the insulin, so the net effect is similar to that of IDD, namely not enough insulin action on the tissues. People with NIDD are often overweight at diagnosis and sometimes slimming is all that is required to control the diabetes. This form of diabetes is often treated by diet alone, though in many cases tablets are also prescribed to boost the body's insulin production.

There is no clear-cut division between people with or without diabetes; there is a continuous spectrum. Thus some people may have a diabetic type of metabolism (body chemistry), but not sufficiently so for the clinical signs of diabetes to be obvious. They are of the non-insulin-dependent type: they produce insulin, but it does not work properly. These 'borderline diabetics', of which there are about three million in the UK, may perhaps get symptoms from time to time, during stress, pregnancy or periods of overweight, for example, but the symptoms disappear again when all is normal. Even so, their diabetic tendency puts them at a disadvantage in respect of coronary heart disease to which both diabetics and borderline diabetics are prone.

Obesity

Obesity increases the risk of angina, heart attack and stroke, as well as arthritis and a number of other disagreeable disorders. It is surprising, therefore, that less than half the population in the UK is in the healthy zone for body weight and things are getting worse, as indeed they are in other developed countries. Despite massive media campaigns in recent years, the prevalence of obesity has increased substantially during the past decade.

Thrifty genes

We have emerged only recently from a long history of chronic food shortages. The ability to store food efficiently when it is available is an obvious advantage under such circumstances. And, of course, our energy store is body fat. Equally the ability to conserve calories when they are in short supply is a useful characteristic. And that is how we have evolved – we are good at storing calories as fat and using fat reserves sparingly. We have thrifty genes.

Thrifty genes had survival advantage in the past but that is not what we need now, at least not in developed countries. Indeed thrifty genes have become a disadvantage, even a threat to our health. Everything in life today in Western society favours fat deposition. There is plenty of food available at modest prices. With few exceptions we have more than enough money to buy rich food and alcoholic drink to satisfy our greatest desires, lavish purchases for home consumption, sumptuous eating out and frequent snacking as well.

Reduced calorie expenditure

At the same time as eating our fill we have reduced our calorie expenditure. We have central heating and good clothing to keep warm. We use labour-saving devices at home and in the workplace. We rely on motorized transport, lifts and escalators to move about. In short we are using petroleum energy, electricity, even nuclear power as the equivalent of a food supplement.

Calorie equation

To maintain a trim healthy body line we need to balance calorie input to calorie expenditure. The so-called 'calorie equation' is:

CALORIES CONSUMED = CALORIES USED UP

There is a little leeway if we eat more than we need as the body has the ability to burn off some of the surplus calories we have consumed. The body achieves this masterly feat by building up and breaking down chemicals unnecessarily, a process which uses up calories. It is a form of calorie-wasting.

There are limits to what can be achieved this way. In any case, people with a 'weight problem' often have a rather poor ability as regards calorie burn-off, especially when the excess dietary calories are in the form of fat.

How many people are overweight?

Judging by the number of overweight people (in Britain nearly half the population), a great many people have got their calorie intake and expenditure well out of balance, exceeding the ability of the body to compensate.

As with all of the health problems characteristic of affluent Westernized societies, obesity occurs more commonly in the less well educated and the less well off.

Percentage of people in the UK with a body weight outside the healthy zone

	Men (%)	Women (%)
Underweight	6	9
Normal weight	42	47
Overweight	40	29
Obese	13	16

Source: Based on CHD Statistics, BHF/CPG 1993.

Body-weight management

Overweight does not happen overnight. It is the result of consistently eating more calories than the body uses, over a long period of time. It takes many months, even years, for the excess weight to build up, so do not expect to solve the problem with a few days of crash dieting. You have to accept that it is a job for life to get your calorie balance right. So you need a way of doing it that is agreeable and non-intrusive.

The extent of the obesity varies between individuals. Many people are no more than 'plump' and not at particular health risk unless there are associated problems like diabetes, high blood pressure or high blood cholesterol. But a further 14 per cent are seriously overweight, sufficient for immediate weight reduction to be recommended on health grounds.

These are numbers of epidemic proportions but, strangely, we do not seem overconcerned. We accept obesity as a normal feature of life, perhaps because it is so widespread and so difficult to manage. Perhaps we should not be so complacent. A quick glance at the list of disorders substantially more common in overweight people (above right) should persuade us to take the matter more seriously.

Obesity should be regarded as an illness that needs to be treated. Whether motivated by health or cosmetic considerations, a sound, sensible and effective method of achieving permanent weight control is required.

There is no point in losing weight just to put it back on again. The commitment must be to slim and stay slim. In any case successive bouts of slimming followed by weight gain progressively reduce metabolic rate, making weight reduction even more difficult in the future. You tend to lose muscle and gain body fat and water, becoming feeble and flabby rather than fit and firm. To make matters worse yo-yo slimming actually *increases* the risk of heart attack.

Health problems more frequent in overweight people

Diabetes	Kidney disease
Coronary heart disease	Varicose veins
High blood pressure	Arthritis
Strokes	Piles
Some cancers	Gall stones
Respiratory infection	Surgical risk

Body fat distribution

We are not yet certain about the importance of fat distribution. Fat deposits tend to be higher up (shoulders, waist, stomach) in men and lower down (bottom and thighs) in women. There is growing evidence that coronary risk in men is higher when the fat is deposited in the belly – the 'beer gut'. Measure your waist and your hips, then divide the first measurement by the second to get your waist-hip ratio. A high waist-hip ratio is a disadvantage and should not exceed 1.0 in men or 0.8 in women.

The principle of healthy slimming

Dietary change should be gradual and minimal, even when slimming. Weight loss should be slow and controlled: about 0.5kg/1lb per week is ideal. Special attention needs to be paid to the nutritional quality of your eating when on a reduced calorie intake. There is no point in creating nutrient deficiencies while trying to improve your health by slimming.

Going on a diet is a recipe for failure. Yet this is what nearly all would-be slimmers do. Bookshops are bursting with diet books, magazines overflow with slimming plans, you can buy pills and powders, have injections. But unless at some stage you take charge of your eating and do the planning yourself, you are doomed to fail.

You cannot go on a diet for the rest of your life. If you do go on a diet you will, most likely, be asked to eat unfamiliar foods and be denied your favourite dishes. You will be expected to adopt a meal plan that may not be convenient. And how do you cope if you eat out a lot, perhaps every day in the middle of the day? How do you cope with a cafeteria or restaurant menu if you yourself are not in charge?

If you follow a diet plan, any diet plan, you will lose weight. They have one thing in common: they are all devices to persuade you to consume fewer calories.

When you slim fast, however, it is not only body fat that you lose. On a rigorous diet, body water is lost, giving the impression that true body weight reduction is being achieved. But this is not so. And losing body water upsets the body's electrolyte balance leading to potassium loss, a risky thing to do. When normal eating is resumed, *as inevitably it must be,* the body water is replaced, so there is, inevitably, immediate weight gain. How depressing! And then the fat is replaced as well, if your normal eating pattern is resumed.

So what is the solution? It is to take charge of your eating and do the menu planning yourself. Learn to be an effective diet and lifestyle manager. Modify permanently the eating and living habits which caused the problem in the first place. Take charge of your eating from the outset and design your own weight reduction regime based on your present eating. Deal with the problem once and for all. *The Family Heart Association Guide to Healthy Eating* (page 54) will help you make low-calorie food choices from the foods that you normally eat and enjoy.

Is overweight inherited?

Fat parents often have fat children. Doubtless there is a genetic tendency to fatness in fat families, but inappropriate diet and lifestyle habits acquired during the early years will set the scene for obesity at any time in life and are likely to be the root of the problem.

It is important to get to grips with the problem of overweight in children primarily to instil in them sound dietary and lifestyle practices which will stand them in good stead later in life. The task of weight correction is also easier in growing children than in adults. Calorie restriction can be quite gentle to reduce weight gain, allowing height eventually to catch up with weight – rather than losing weight to match height, which is what adults have to do. Severe crash dieting in children, as in adults, is not a good idea and can interfere with development. Skilful dietary planning, however, can provide a most interesting set of slimming menus to help the child, indeed the whole family, to a healthy body weight. It is within the family that the problem arose, so it is the responsibility of the family to solve it together.

Causes of angina and heart attack

Children respond to obesity in the same way as adults, with a tendency to altered blood glucose regulation, respiratory illness, raised blood pressure and elevated blood cholesterol. But, unsurprisingly, they do not generally suffer, as children, degenerative illnesses such as coronaries, strokes and arthritis; yet they are at increased risk of these disorders in adulthood.

The message is clear: help children by sorting out diet and lifestyle problems when the children are young. Healthy eating and living habits acquired within the family at a young age can, and often do, become the habits of a lifetime.

Assessment of body-weight status

One way to decide about the amount of fat on your body is to look objectively in a mirror. Do not be put off by a little plumpness. Stand tall and proud. Dress well. Believe in yourself. But ask yourself honestly – is it more than plumpness? Perhaps you should examine your eating anyway; a small amount of overweight is an early warning that something is not quite right in the balance of your eating and living. Overweight is easier to remedy when the problem is a small one.

To assess your body weight status, refer to the chart on page 27. You can, if you prefer,

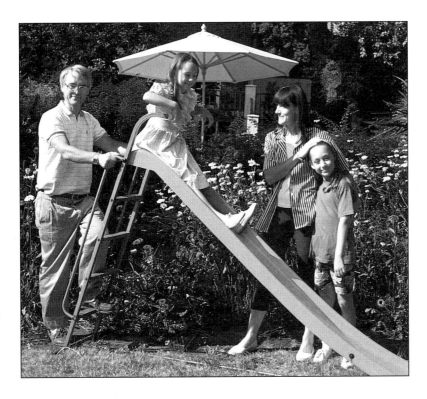

When both parents are fat, the chance of overweight in the children is high, but when both parents are lean, the risk falls.

take a more scientific approach to body weight assessment and calculate your body mass index (BMI), which is the best and most widely used indicator of excess body weight. Here is the formula:

$$\text{Body mass index} = \frac{\text{Weight (kg)}}{\text{Height (m)}^2}$$

If you know your height only in inches and your weight in pounds, the formula then becomes:

$$\text{Body mass index} = \frac{\text{Weight (lb)} \times 700}{\text{Height (in)}^2}$$

To assess your body weight compare against the reference values in the table (above right).

Body mass index	Category
Less than 17.5	Too thin
17.5–20.0	Borderline thin
20.0–25.0	Healthy zone
25.0–27.5	Borderline fat
27.5–30.0	Too fat
More than 30.0	Obese

Another way to find out whether you are in the healthy zone for body weight is from the table on page 28.

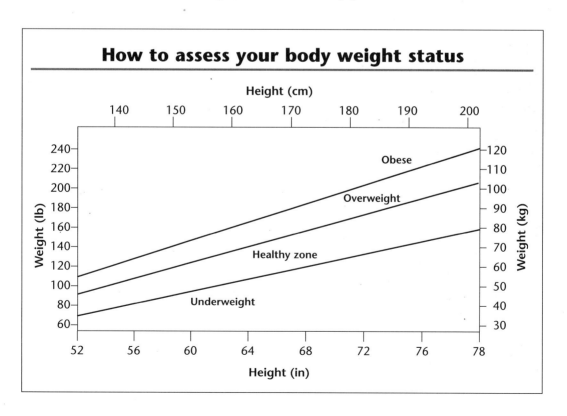

How to assess your body weight status

Causes of angina and heart attack

Healthy body weight range		
Height ft in	**Weight (lb) BMI 20**	**Weight (lb) BMI 25**
4 6	83	104
8	90	112
10	96	120
5 0	103	129
2	110	137
4	117	146
6	125	156
8	132	165
10	140	175
6 0	148	185
2	157	196
4	165	206
6	174	217

Height cm	**Weight (kg) BMI 20**	**Weight (kg) BMI 25**
140	39	49
145	42	53
150	45	56
155	48	60
160	51	64
165	55	68
170	58	72
175	61	77
180	65	81
185	68	86
190	72	90
195	76	95
200	80	100

If your BMI is more than 25, you should plan to lose some weight. At 25 to 27.5 you are borderline overweight, a little plump.

If your BMI is more than 27.5, you are strongly advised to lose some weight and to examine your diet and lifestyle generally. What is causing the problem? What is the best way to deal with it?

If your BMI is in excess of 30 there can be no delay or indecision. To lose some weight is essential, a medical necessity. If you are very heavily muscled, a body builder or weight lifter perhaps, your BMI may be a bit high without an excess of fat. But do not delude yourself. Very few people are in that category.

The elderly tend to a lower BMI because inactivity leads to loss of muscle tissue. They should be encouraged to exercise any muscles they can to stop them wasting away. Apart from anything else, having more muscle helps to keep you warm – muscle generates more metabolic heat than fat.

Why activity is helpful to slimmers

It is helpful to remain physically active while slimming, and as an aid to weight management generally. There are several reasons for this. When your calorie intake decreases, your body responds by trying to save every calorie it can. It shuts down the fat stores you are keen to use up. It makes you lethargic so that you do not burn up calories unnecessarily.

If you are active, however, the body responds in the opposite way. It responds as if your life is threatened and you need to run away or defend yourself, the so-called 'fight or flight' reaction. The fat stores are opened up to help provide the necessary fuel. The circulation flows freely and you are ready for action. Despite a reduced calorie intake your body will expend calories in the interest of survival. Quite apart from any calories that may be used up by the exercise itself, the body metabolism becomes more 'spendthrift' and slimming is made easier. In short, physical activity puts your body into a calorie burn-up mode.

As a bonus, of course, exercise tones up your muscles and improves your circulation, so you feel good and look good too. Muscles use more calories than fat tissue, so replacing some of your excess fat with a bit of extra muscle will make it easier to stay slim for life.

But what sort of exercise is required?

You do not need to torture yourself in a gymnasium or aerobics class – if you find it torture, that is; some people enjoy such activities. Brisk walking, swimming, cycling, gardening, dancing are all good exercise. So are home exercises, doing the housework or car cleaning vigorously, using the stairs instead of the lift – walking upstairs or uphill is really quite a strenuous activity. There are many ways to add a little activity into your life. See how many ways you can find to do that.

Regular physical activity in the battle against obesity is also good for diabetes and reduces the risk of coronary heart disease. Regular suitable exercise is part of the treatment for people with angina and for those who have survived a heart attack. However, before embarking on a programme of physical activity, it is desirable to go through a warm-up routine.

Athletes and professional sportsmen do this because it reduces the chance of strains and sprains, damage to tendons, ligaments and joints. You should do it too, even before something as basic as a 'training walk'. And after your 'training' exercise, do the warm-up routine again. The gentle stretching reduces the chance of aches and pains the next day. The warm-up routine also has merit in its own right, to improve general suppleness.

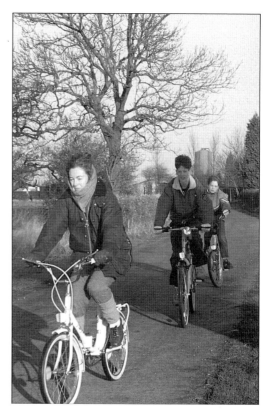

You do not have to go to the gym to exercise. Try cycling.

Causes of angina and heart attack

Warm-up exercises

Whatever your present level of fitness, you should begin and finish any period of exercise with the following stretching exercises.

Then, when you have finished your training exercises, have a nice warm bath, a change of clothes and a contented feeling of achievement.

Lower leg stretch

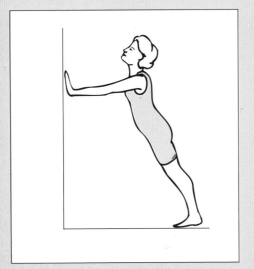

Stand upright about 1m/3ft from a wall or post. Keeping the feet apart and flat on the floor or ground, extend the arms forward, hands flat on the wall, and lean forward. Hold that position for five seconds, feeling the tension in the back of the calves and upper legs. Straighten up and rest for five seconds. Repeat the exercise ten times.

Lower back and buttock stretch

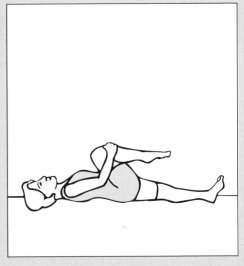

Lie on your back and bring one knee up and into the chest, pulling the knee as far forward as possible and feeling the stretch in your back and buttock. Hold the position for five seconds, then rest for five seconds. Then do the same with the other leg. Repeat this procedure ten times with each leg.

Back extension

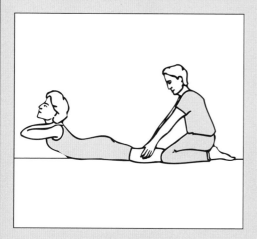

Lie flat on your front. Arch your back and hold for five seconds. This exercise is made easier if a partner holds your legs down or if you hook your heels under a heavy piece of furniture. Repeat ten times.

Upper body rotation for back, side and shoulder

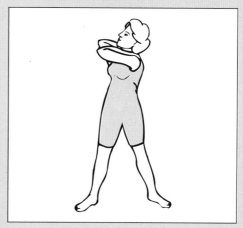

Stand upright, hands behind the head, feet astride. While remaining vertical, rotate the trunk as far as possible first to the left, then to the right. Repeat ten times in each direction.

Hip rotation for hips and back

Stand upright, hands on hips and feet astride. Bending from the waist, lean to the left, then rotate forwards and to the right, thence returning to the upright position. Repeat ten times in each direction.

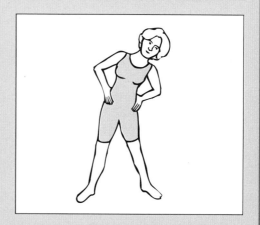

Causes of angina and heart attack

Head rotation
for neck and upper back

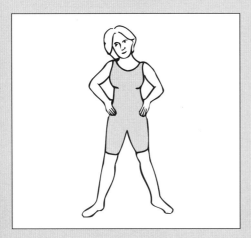

Stand upright, hands on hips and feet astride. Slowly and gently rotate the head clockwise in a full circle ten times. Then anti-clockwise ten times.

Head and shoulder curl for
neck and upper back

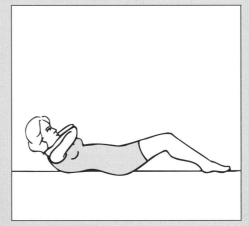

Lie flat on your back, hands behind your head. Slowly curl the head forward, lifting the shoulders off the ground. Hold for five seconds. Rest for five seconds. Repeat ten times.

Upper body pike
for hamstrings and
lower back

Sit on the floor, legs straight, with the back of the knees pressed flat on the floor. Grasp under the knees and slowly pull the body forward and down towards the knees. Hold for five seconds. Sit upright again, rest for five seconds. Repeat ten times.

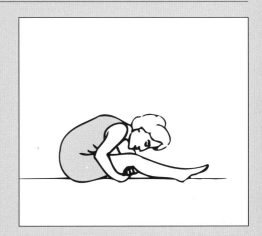

Remember that these are gentle stretching exercises, not training exercises. Even top athletes go through a warm-up and cool-down routine when training or performing, so you are in good company.

And before you move into your full exercise routine, get your heart and circulation loosened up too by walking, slowly at first, then more and more briskly for at least five minutes – until you are thoroughly warm. After the training session walk for five minutes progressively more slowly to prevent the circulation having to adapt abruptly from going flat out to being at baseline level again. Stopping abruptly leads to pooling of blood in the legs and unpleasant feelings of faintness, dizziness and discomfort.

If you are very out of condition, you would do well to spend a few weeks doing just the warm-up stretching exercises, the five-minute warm-up walk, then a ten-minute brisk training walk, as fast as you comfortably can, followed by a five-minute cool-down walk and then the stretching exercises again, but this time to 'ease down'.

Heart risk questionnaire

Detailed questionnaires with graded responses and scores are often misleading, so we have devised a simpler, more useful one. If you answer 'yes' to *any* of the questions below, you need a check-up by your doctor

1   Do you have a close (blood) relative who had angina or a heart attack below the age of 60?

2   Do you suffer regular chest pains, especially after exertion such as going upstairs or hurrying for a bus? This pain may or may not be accompanied by undue breathlessness.

3   Do you have thickening of the Achilles tendon at the back of the ankles, lumps on the knuckles or yellowish patches around the eyes? (See the pictures on page 18.)

4   Do you have a close (blood) relative with high blood cholesterol?

5   Do you know if your blood pressure is elevated?

6   Do you have a close (blood) relative with high blood pressure?

7   Do you have to urinate frequently and are you always thirsty? This could indicate a diabetic tendency which might increase the risk of developing coronary heart disease.

Chapter four
Medical treatments

Angina

Angina, which is also called angina pectoris, is the name for the severe but temporary chest pain which is caused by an inadequate supply of oxygen to the heart muscle. Pain is usually felt in the middle of the chest, but may spread to the neck or jaw or across a shoulder and down an arm. Occasionally the pain may occur over the stomach or between the shoulder blades. Words often used by sufferers to describe the pain include: tightness, heaviness, pressure, bursting, tight band, constriction, pain, discomfort and weight on the chest.

Angina occurs in two forms: it may be 'stable' or 'unstable'.

Stable angina

Stable angina is predictable; it comes on after a known amount of exercise. The severity is usually the same each time and is relieved by the same amount of rest or the usual dose of medication. It does not occur at rest and will not wake you at night.

Unstable angina

Unstable angina is not relieved by usual doses of medication. It occurs after progressively less exercise and may occur at rest or wake you up at night. It is more serious than stable angina and may be followed by a heart attack. If you have angina which is not relieved by your usual medication, you should contact your doctor or call for an ambulance.

Diagnosis of angina by your family doctor

The doctor will carry out a full examination, including listening to your heart and chest, looking at your hands and feet for swelling and to check the circulation.

Your height, weight and blood pressure will be measured and the doctor will look for physical signs of a high blood cholesterol, such as a white ring around the coloured part of the eye (this is a sign only in younger patients, under 50; older people may develop a similar white ring as a normal part of ageing), and lumps on the Achilles tendons of the heels and on the knuckles or backs of the hands (see pages 18).

A blood sample will be taken and tested for cholesterol and triglyceride (another blood fat), and blood glucose will be measured to check for diabetes. A full blood count may also be carried out to check for anaemia, which can make the symptoms of angina worse. You will be asked to starve overnight before the test.

An electrocardiogram (ECG) is usually carried out. The result generally is normal in angina when taken at rest, but may show abnormalities during an exercise test (see page 36). An electrode is attached to each of your arms and legs and some are also attached to your chest. Wires are connected to the electrodes and these are plugged into a machine which can detect the beats or

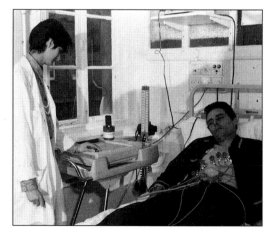

A patient undergoing an ECG.

electrical activity of the heart. This activity is then recorded on to paper. The process is completely painless.

The ECG is used to detect any abnormalities in the way the heart is beating. It can detect both recent and older heart attacks and can also tell the doctor if the heart is enlarged or under strain. Occasionally you may also have a chest X-ray.

Hospital tests
Some tests are carried out in hospital as more specialized equipment is needed.

Exercise ECG
One test which may be done in hospital is an exercise ECG. This is an ECG which is carried out while you are on an exercise treadmill or an exercise bicycle. It is a helpful test if you suffer from angina when exercising but feel perfectly well when you are resting. The ECG can be recorded while you are experiencing the symptoms of angina. Sometimes your doctor may ask you to stop taking some of your heart medication for a couple of days before the test. You will need to wear comfortable shoes and loose comfortable clothing. Your blood pressure will be checked regularly during the test, and a doctor will be present.

The test begins with easy gentle exercise, which is gradually made more difficult. The test stops when you become tired, short of breath, if the ECG changes, your chest pain gets worse or the heart rate reaches the set target. The ECG is recorded during the exercise and continues for a few minutes after you have stopped. The test takes about fifteen minutes and you will probably find that it is hard work, but you may be surprised to see just how much you can achieve.

If the ECG changes at the same time as you suffer from chest pain, this usually indicates that the pain is coming from the heart. ECG changes and chest pain which happen at a low level of exercise are usually more serious than if they occur at a high level of exercise, and further tests may be carried out.

Medical treatments

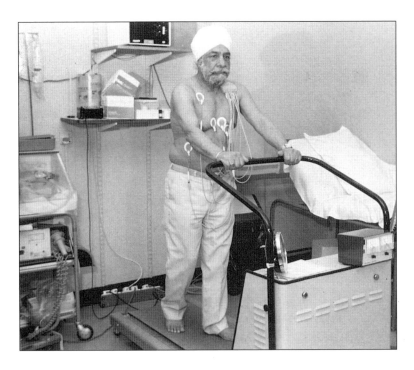

An exercise ECG is a helpful test for patients who suffer from angina when exercising but who feel perfectly well when resting.

Exercise ECGs are sometimes carried out after a heart attack, but you would not be asked to exercise quite as hard. Such a test is useful after a heart attack as it can give you the confidence to begin to exercise at a time when many people fear that exercise will cause another heart attack. A programme of gradually increasing exercise is actually part of the treatment for heart attack once the crisis is over.

Twenty-four-hour tape recording of the ECG

The ECG can also be recorded over 24 hours. This test is usually done out of hospital and is used to record the ECG if you suffer symptoms such as palpitations which you may not get regularly. You will have to visit the hospital twice, once to be attached to the recorder and again for it to be removed. Leads will be attached to your chest, and these feed into a small box which you wear around your waist attached to a belt. You then carry on with your usual daily activities (apart from having a bath or shower). You will be given a diary to complete for the day, to record any symptoms you experience along with the time they occur. It is important that you complete this as accurately as possible. The diary can then be compared with the ECG.

Echocardiography

Echocardiography is the same technique which is used to look at the developing baby in pregnant women, when it is often called a

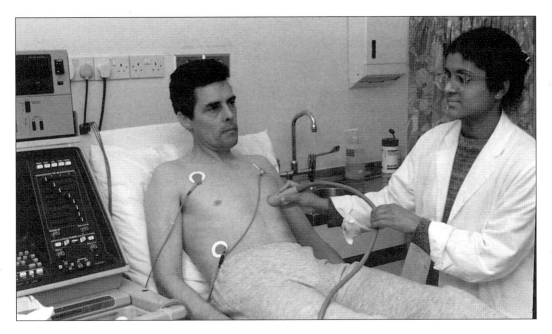

Echocardiography in progress.

scan. A probe is placed on the chest wall and sound waves are transmitted from the probe into the chest. The sound waves are reflected from the heart and picked up by the probe and are then shown on a screen as a picture. The speed of blood flow through the heart can also be measured (a process known as Doppler echocardiography). The test can take up to an hour to carry out, but is harmless and totally painless.

Radionuclide test

The radionuclide test is very specialized and rarely carried out. A radioactive substance called an isotope is injected into a vein, sometimes while you are exercising. A special camera can then be used to look at the heart as

it fills with blood and empties, and to look at the blood flow through the arteries which supply the heart. The dose of radiation is very small and compares to that which you would get from a chest X-ray.

Cardiac catheterization

Cardiac catheterization is a test which has several uses. It can be carried out to measure the blood pressure in the heart, to look at the chambers and valves of the heart, or to look at the coronary arteries to check where the blockages are within them. For this test you may need to stay overnight in hospital, or you may need to stay for just a short time after the catheterization. Before the test is carried out you will need to have an empty stomach and

Medical treatments

you may be given a 'premed' injection or tablet. Cardiac catheterization is carried out in an X-ray room and will take between 20 minutes and one hour to complete.

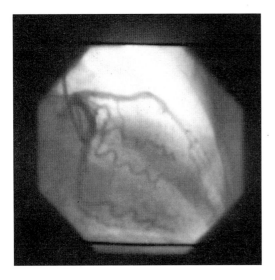

X-ray showing the arteries which supply the heart with blood.

What does this involve?
The catheter is a very narrow, very flexible plastic tube about 1m/3ft long. The skin where the catheter is to be inserted is injected with local anaesthetic to numb it. The injection will sting a little, but after that you will not feel anything. The catheter is inserted into either an artery or a vein, either at the groin or in an arm through a small cut in the skin. It is then fed through the artery or vein until it reaches the heart. The doctor does this by using X-rays to help place the catheter in the correct position in the heart. You can watch the

procedure on the X-ray screen if you wish. You will not be able to feel the catheter moving inside you, but you may be aware of an occasional 'missed' heart beat. When the catheter is in the correct place, fluid is injected into it. This fluid will show up on the X-ray film (see the photograph on the left). As the fluid is injected, pictures are taken. You may feel a hot sensation as the fluid is injected. Some people may have an angina pain, and you should tell the doctor if this happens – it does not mean that something has gone wrong. During the procedure the blood pressure is taken at the tip of the catheter and an ECG (recording of your heart beat) is monitored continuously.

After the test is completed and the catheter is removed, either a few stitches are needed in the arm, or pressure is applied over the groin for about ten minutes to prevent bleeding and reduce bruising. You may feel tired for a few hours after the test. Your arm or groin will be checked after the test at intervals to make sure that the wound does not bleed.

Is there any risk attached to cardiac catheterization?
This is now a common procedure and complications are rare. Occasionally you will get a bruise where the catheter was inserted at the groin, or the pulse in the arm will become weaker. These are not serious, but the bruising will probably be sore for a few days.

More serious problems are rare. About one in 700 people will have a heart attack during the test. Cardiac catheterization is not carried out, however, unless the benefit of the test

38

outweighs the risk. If you are worried about this, talk to your doctor before you undergo the test.

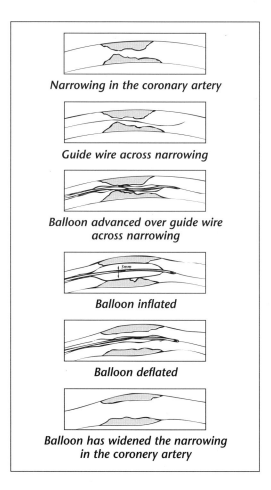

Narrowing in the coronary artery

Guide wire across narrowing

Balloon advanced over guide wire across narrowing

↕ 3mm

Balloon inflated

Balloon deflated

Balloon has widened the narrowing in the coronery artery

Coronary angioplasty

Coronary angioplasty was first carried out in 1977, so is a relatively new way of treating coronary artery disease. The procedure is similar to cardiac catheterization but this time a small balloon is attached to the end of the catheter. The balloon is positioned in the blocked or narrowed coronary artery and it is then inflated, so stretching the artery and compressing the material (plaque) which is causing the blockage. The balloon is then deflated and removed, leaving a wider artery which allows more blood to pass through to the heart muscle. The angioplasty takes longer to carry out than cardiac catheterization as it is a more complicated procedure. Many people get angina pains during the angioplasty, but these improve when the balloon is deflated.

Can everyone with angina have angioplasty?
Unfortunately only about one third of patients who have cardiac catheterization are suitable for angioplasty. Often there are too many blockages, or the blockage is too tight or too long for current technology to cope with.

People who have had coronary bypass graft surgery (see page 40) can sometimes have angioplasty if the graft becomes narrowed.

Are there any risks?
Angioplasty usually takes place without any problems. Occasionally, however, it causes complete blockage of the artery which the doctor has been trying to widen, or the artery may tear. The doctor may think that this will lead to serious damage to the heart and ask a surgeon to operate and carry out a coronary artery bypass graft to reduce the damage.

If you are about to have angioplasty, you should therefore be prepared for the slight chance that you may need further *immediate* surgery. This happens to a maximum of one in every 75 patients treated.

Medical treatments

The angioplasty may be unsuccessful and you may then need to be referred for surgery and placed on the waiting list. The doctor will explain this to you.

Can the arteries block again?
Angina recurs in around one in five people who have an angioplasty. Angioplasty can often be repeated successfully. If angina has not recurred after six months, recurrence is unusual. Some patients who were treated over ten years ago are still free from the pain of angina.

Does angioplasty have advantages over bypass surgery?
Yes, if you are suitable for this treatment. If you have angioplasty, you will need a shorter hospital stay as the procedure does not involve major surgery. You will need less time off work, and the angioplasty can usually be repeated if the artery reblocks. Angioplasty can occasionally be used to treat people who cannot have major surgery.

Are there any other treatments?
Research is going on all the time to improve the treatment of people who are suffering from coronary heart disease.
● Lasers are being used to unblock arteries. This treatment is not widely available at the moment and very few people are suitable.
● A device which rotates, similar to a drill, can be fed through the catheter to remove the material which is causing the blockage.
● Small metal coils called stents can be placed in the artery and expanded to hold the artery open.
● The blockage can sometimes be broken up using ultrasound energy.

New advances are being made all the time. Contact the British Heart Foundation (at the address on page 79) to find out about the latest developments.

Coronary artery bypass graft surgery
Coronary artery bypass surgery is carried out when one or more of the coronary arteries is blocked and cannot be unblocked by angioplasty. A new passageway is created for the blood to pass through to restore the blood flow to the heart muscle at the other end of the blockage. This is in the same way that traffic

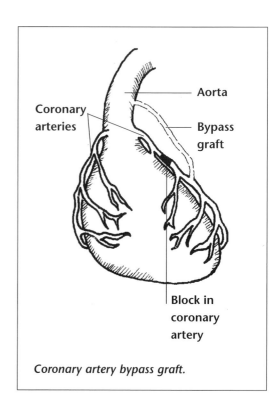

Coronary arteries

Aorta

Bypass graft

Block in coronary artery

Coronary artery bypass graft.

bypasses a congested city or town centre by using an alternative road. Blood is diverted from the main blood vessel coming out of the heart, an artery called the aorta, to the other side of the blockage. A new route, known as a graft, is created for each of the arteries which is blocked or narrowed. You may need only one new route or graft, but more often people need two, three or four; these are called double, triple and quadruple by-passes.

How is this done?
A blood vessel is taken from another part of your body to form the graft – usually an artery from inside the chest wall. If, for some reason, these arteries are not suitable, a vein may be used, usually from a leg. If you have had varicose vein surgery, these veins may not be suitable, in which case a vein will be taken from an arm to form the graft.

The surgeon carries out the operation through a cut made in the front of the chest. The bone which is in front of the heart (the breast bone or sternum) has to be cut to allow the surgeon to get to the heart. While the heart is being operated on, it has to be stopped, which means that blood is no longer passing through the heart, lungs or rest of the body. A heart/lung bypass machine is used to take over the job of the heart and lungs; this oxygenates the blood and pumps it around the body.

How long will it take me to recover from surgery?
You will probably be in hospital for about two weeks: usually for two or three days before the operation and about nine to ten days after.

Most people take about three months to recover fully from heart surgery, but this time varies according to the individual. Remember that the breast bone has been cut in two during the surgery and takes a while to heal, sometimes many weeks. You may have muscular pain in the centre of the chest, neck, back and arms: this is normal after this type of surgery, and you should see your doctor for advice on pain relief.

Some people also have feelings of numbness or pins and needles around the scar in the leg or arm if a vein has been used for the graft, but this again is normal and need not be worried about. You may find that your leg swells and you may have to wear an elastic stocking on the leg for a few weeks when you are sitting at home. Try keeping your leg elevated when you are sitting.

Some people can feel depressed after the surgery; however, this is a normal reaction after any major surgery. You may also feel anxious, particularly when you arrive home. You will feel better on some days than others.

Try some of the relaxation techniques described from page 73 onwards. If you are reading this before you have surgery, relaxation may also help prior to the operation when you may be feeling understandably anxious.

If you are feeling depressed and are finding it difficult to cope, talk to your doctor, who will be able to help you.

Can I go back to work?
Most people are able to return to their previous job after bypass surgery. Between 75 and 85 per cent of people go back to their

Medical treatments

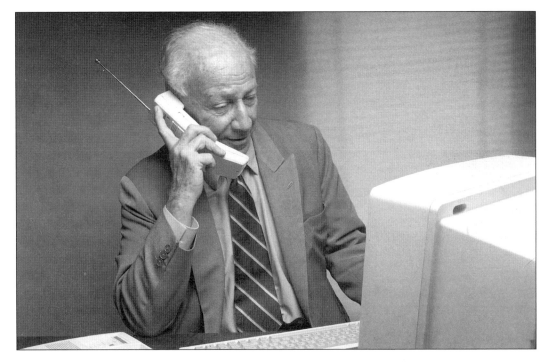

Most people are fit enough to return to their previous job after bypass surgery.

previous employment. If you have a light occupation, you will be able to return to work earlier than if you have a job which involves more manual work. People in lighter occupations may be able to go back to work after about two months. If your job involves heavy manual work, you will need to wait longer to give the chest wall longer to heal, usually at least three months.

What about sex?

You should be able to resume sexual intercourse after about four weeks, but be careful not to place too much stress on your chest wound or to restrict your breathing.

Can I drive again?

If you feel fit enough, you can begin to drive a car again after about six weeks. You need to inform your insurance company; there may be restrictions which apply to you.

Is the surgery effective?

Most people – up to 80 per cent – who have a coronary artery bypass graft will be free from angina pain and the pain relief is long-lasting. In most of the rest of people who undergo the operation, the pain will be improved. In some people complete pain relief will not be possible, but the operation will be worthwhile if the level of pain can be reduced.

What are the risks?

Obviously there are risks attached to any major surgery such as coronary bypass surgery. Around one to two people out of every 100 die within 30 days of the operation. This is a very low rate in public health terms and shows how successful this type of surgery is. If you have had major heart attacks which have damaged the heart muscle, the risk will be greater than for someone with less damage.

Can I do anything to help myself?

You can certainly do things to help yourself.

You must give up smoking. If you have not already stopped, you must stop now. See page 68 for help with this. If you carry on, you will double the chances of the graft blocking again.

See page 53 for advice on diet, page 29 for exercise suggestions, page 23 for body weight and page 64 for alcohol consumption.

Can coronary heart disease be cured?

A question often asked is whether all the coronary arteries are likely to be blocked. Usually it is only one artery or parts of the arteries which have become blocked by the fatty deposits. In some people the blood supply finds a new way around the blockage.

Eating a diet which is low in fat may help to reduce the narrowing. There are also cholesterol-lowering drugs which may help, or the narrowing can be corrected by inserting a balloon into the blockage and inflating it (see page 39). Some people need to have an operation which bypasses the blockage and provides the heart with a new blood supply.

The heart and its recovery from a heart attack

The heart has amazing powers of recovery. The amount of recovery it makes depends on how much of the heart muscle has died following a heart attack. The rest of the heart will take over the work of the damaged part. Taking regular exercise will help to strengthen the heart muscle further and speed up the healing process. Build up gently after the heart attack. Many people become fitter after their heart attack than they were before because they begin to look after themselves better.

When recovering from a heart attack, you will find that you have time to reflect on healthy changes you can make to your diet and lifestyle.

What to do in an emergency

Everyone should know what to do in an emergency. You may never need to use this information, but it is better to be prepared than sorry. Get everyone who lives with you to read this section or, even better, you might choose to go on a life-saving course run by the Red Cross or the St John Ambulance (addresses on page 79).

Medical treatments

What to do if you think that you are having a heart attack

A heart attack should always be treated as an emergency, as the beating of the heart can be disturbed or even stop. Treatment with drugs to dissolve the clot needs to be started as soon as possible after the heart attack. You could place an aspirin under your tongue, to be sucked slowly, unless you have been told by your doctor not to take aspirin. Tell the ambulance person if you have done this.

What are the symptoms of a heart attack?
- A crushing vice-like pain in the chest. The pain may spread down the left arm or both arms or into the throat and jaw.
- The skin will be white and the nail beds and lips may look blue.
- You may feel cold, faint, dizzy, sick, clammy.

What to do
- If the pain is bearable, try to relax. If you have been given tablets or a spray for angina by your doctor, use them. If the pain goes away, it may have been angina.
- If the pain has not lessened within 20 minutes of taking angina medication, treat it as a heart attack.

Suspected heart attack
- If the pain is unbearable, phone your doctor and explain what your symptoms are.
- If you cannot contact your doctor after five minutes, or if the doctor is on the way and the pain becomes much worse, or if the doctor is on the way but you feel about to pass out, dial 999 and ask for an ambulance. Tell them that you think you are having a heart attack.
- If you cannot get to a phone, ask someone to drive you to the nearest hospital. *Do not drive yourself.*
- While you are waiting, unlock the door to the house if you can. Lie on your side and wait for the doctor or ambulance.
- Always keep your doctor's telephone number by the phone, so that you can easily find it in an emergency.

What to do if someone collapses

First you must call for help. Dial 999, ask for an ambulance and tell them what has happened. If someone else is with you, get them to do this. If you are alone, call for help before trying to aid the collapsed person.

If the heart has stopped beating, the person will lose consciousness very quickly and may stop breathing. In this case you will not be able to find a pulse.

Resuscitation
Before you do anything you must first assess the situation. Run through this ABC of checks:
- **A = Airway** Check that the airway is clear of obstructions and remove loose or badly fitting dentures.
- **B = Breathing** Assess the airway by holding your hand or cheek just in front of the casualty's mouth to feel for breath. Listen for breath sounds and look for chest movements.
- **C = Circulation** Feel for the carotid pulse in the neck, next to the windpipe. Feel for it on yourself so that you know what you are looking for. If there is no pulse, you must begin cardiac massage immediately.

The brain can survive for only two to four minutes unless resuscitation is started immediately. Place the casualty on a firm surface, lying on their back, and ensure that the airway is clear. Tilt the head back, extending the neck, which will open the airway.

Pinch the nose to seal it, take a deep breath, place your mouth over the casualty's mouth to make a seal and breathe out (see the illustration on page 46). Watch that the casualty's chest rises as you breathe out: this will tell you that you are doing this right. Allow the breath to escape from the mouth and watch the chest fall. Repeat.

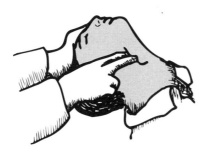

Finding the carotid pulse

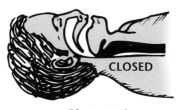

Obstructed

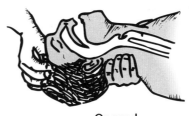

Opened

Extending the neck to open the airway.

Medical treatments

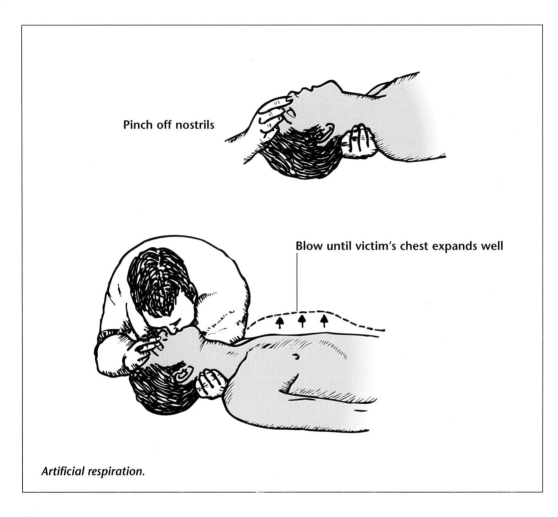

Pinch off nostrils

Blow until victim's chest expands well

Artificial respiration.

With one finger feel for the edge of the bone which joins both sets of ribs, place the heel of the other hand just above the finger so it is on the sternum, the bone between the ribs. Place your first hand on top of this hand. Keep your arms straight, and lean forward to compress the chest by about 5 cm/2 in.

If you are on your own, do two breaths followed by 15 chest compressions. If there are two of you, do one breath to five chest compressions. Continue until the ambulance arrives.

If the casualty recovers before the ambulance arrives (begins breathing without assistance and the pulse returns), lay them on their side and check at frequent intervals that they are breathing and have a pulse.

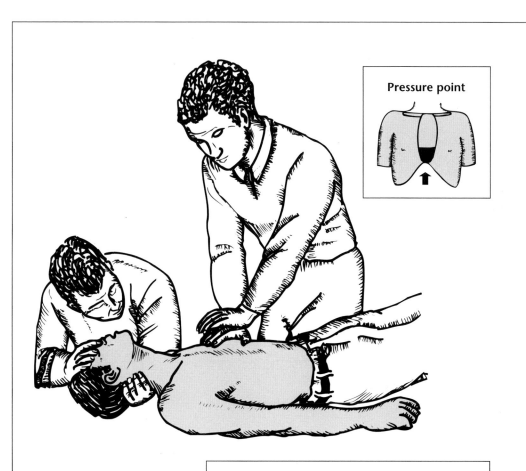

Pressure point

Heel of hand on pressure point

Other hand on
top of first

DO NOT ALLOW FINGERS
TO TOUCH CHEST WALL!

Cardiac massage.

Chapter five

Drug treatments

Cardiac drugs

This section contains information on some of the more commonly used cardiac drugs. For further information speak to your doctor or pharmacist.

If you have been prescribed drugs, it is important that you take them *as they have been prescribed*. Write down their names and keep a list of them with you. This will be very useful if you need to see a new doctor or are admitted to hospital unexpectedly. If you feel that you do not want to take the drugs or think that you are experiencing side effects, discuss this with your doctor – *do not* just stop taking them as this could be dangerous.

Modern drugs are very safe, but most drugs have some side effects. Serious side effects are very rare, but minor ones are more common. If you do think that you are experiencing any side effects, tell your doctor, who may need to prescribe a different drug or simply adjust the dose.

If you forget which tablet you have to take when, try writing a list. You will soon get into the habit of taking them. If this does not help, speak to your doctor, as there are special containers available to help you with the problem.

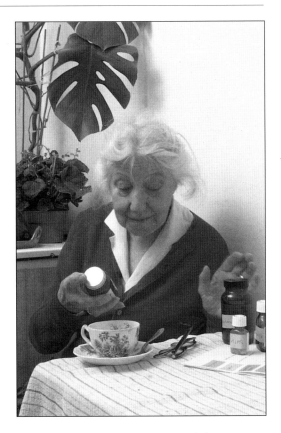

If you have been prescribed several drugs and forget which tablet to take when, try writing a list.

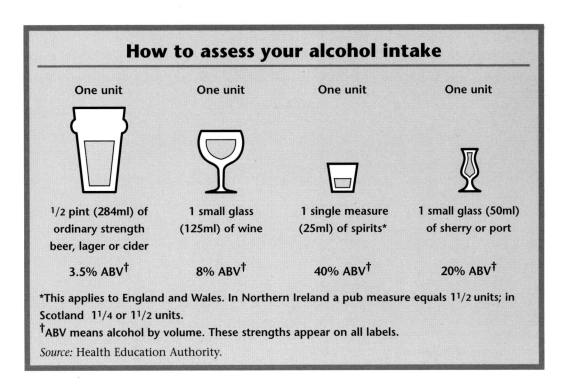

How to assess your alcohol intake

One unit	One unit	One unit	One unit
1/2 pint (284ml) of ordinary strength beer, lager or cider	1 small glass (125ml) of wine	1 single measure (25ml) of spirits*	1 small glass (50ml) of sherry or port
3.5% ABV[†]	8% ABV[†]	40% ABV[†]	20% ABV[†]

*This applies to England and Wales. In Northern Ireland a pub measure equals 1¹/2 units; in Scotland 1¹/4 or 1¹/2 units.

[†]ABV means alcohol by volume. These strengths appear on all labels.

Source: Health Education Authority.

High cholesterol

Survivors of heart attack are at particularly high risk of further attacks and will benefit most from reducing the cholesterol and other fats in the blood. Blood fats should be measured within 24 hours of a heart attack as there is often a fall in plasma cholesterol levels over the next three months as a result of the attack which gives a false impression of the true situation.

Management of high cholesterol

If you have high cholesterol, you will first be given dietary advice which aims to reduce your intake of saturated fats (see page 59). When you have kept to this diet for three to six months, another blood test will be carried out which will measure total cholesterol, high-density lipoprotein, low-density lipoprotein, and triglycerides; you will need to fast for this test for between 12 and 14 hours. Ideally total cholesterol should be lowered to less than 5.2 mmol/l and LDL to less than 3.4 mmol/l following a heart attack. LDL cholesterol in people who have not had a heart attack should be less than 4.1 mmol/l. The target for the 'good' cholesterol, HDL, is above 1 mmol/l.

How can what I eat help?

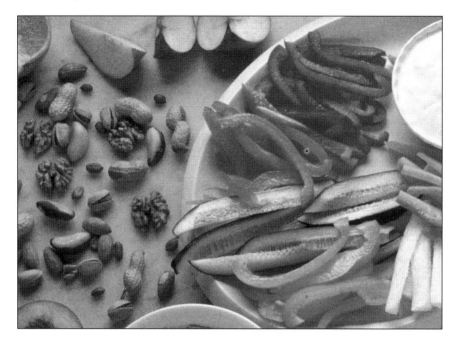

Try these foods for healthier snacks: vegetable sticks, fresh and dried fruit, a few nuts, and cereals.

Triglycerides

High blood triglyceride levels are often associated with obesity, a sedentary lifestyle, high blood pressure, high alcohol intake, a high level of sugar intake and diabetes. These should all be controlled before treating a high triglyceride level, but if the triglycerides remain over 2.3 mmol/l, drug treatment should be considered, especially if this occurs in association with a high blood cholesterol.

Cutting down on sugar

● If you want something sweet to eat, try looking in the fruit bowl rather than the biscuit barrel. Fruit will also provide you with vitamins, minerals and fibre.

● Try using dried fruit to sweeten milk puddings, cakes and sauces.

● Look at the labels on foods that you buy to check for added sugar. Canned vegetables and soups can have sugar added.

● Sugary fruit drinks, squashes and fizzy drinks can be packed with sugar. An average can of cola contains about eight teaspoons of sugar.

● Buy canned fruits in juice rather than in syrup.

● You can buy reduced-sugar jams and sugar-free fruit spreads. Try using pear and apple spread as a sugar substitute in baking.

● Look out for sugar on food labels. 'Healthy' biscuit-type bars, for example, are often higher in sugar that you think. Check labels for sucrose, glucose, dextrose, fructose (fruit sugar), invert sugars and syrup – they are all sugars.

Watch out for hidden fats

Cakes and biscuits, particularly when shop-bought, can be very high in saturated fat as well as in calories. You can make your own cakes and biscuits with polyunsaturated or monounsaturated fat – they will be even more tasty if home-made. Try adapting your own recipes by substituting 75ml/5 tablespoons of vegetable oil for each 100g/4oz of margarine or butter. If you need to reduce your intake of dietary cholesterol, try using just egg white (this does not contain any cholesterol) in recipes rather than the whole egg, or replace each egg with 30ml/2 tablespoons of milk.

If you have high triglycerides, you will need to avoid cakes, biscuits and chocolate as these are high in sugar. Some food manufacturers are now producing cakes which are low in fat (look out for these in the supermarkets), but remember that they are high in sugar so need to be eaten in moderation, especially if you are trying to lose weight or reduce your triglycerides.

In summary, eat a varied diet. Eat plenty of vegetables, fruits and starchy foods such as bread, potatoes, rice and pasta. Reduce your intake of fat, especially saturated fats, and foods which are high in sugar and salt. Drink alcohol in modest amounts. But most of all enjoy your food.

For more information about diet ask your doctor to refer you to a dietitian, or contact the Family Heart Association (address on page 79).

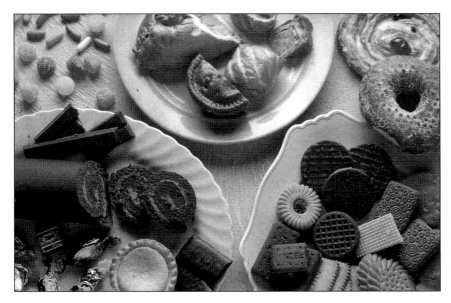

Go easy on cakes, biscuits, chocolates and sweets, which tend to be high in fat.

Chapter seven

Smoking, body weight and stress

Smoking and lifestyle

Stopping smoking is probably the most important contribution you can make to your recovery. If you stop smoking, you are twice as likely to see the fifth anniversary of your heart attack than if you continue to smoke. The risk of your having another heart attack in your first year will be halved.

Stopping smoking will also reduce your chances of developing other diseases associated with smoking such as lung and other cancers, bronchitis and so on.

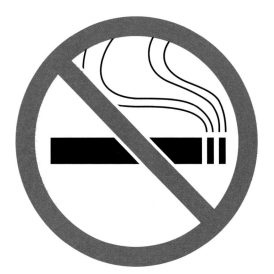

How to give up smoking

Giving up smoking is as difficult as getting off heroin; the nicotine in cigarettes is very addictive. Giving up smoking will take a lot of willpower and determination, but it will be worth it.

How to avoid having 'just one cigarette'

Each time you refuse to have a cigarette, you will be extending your life. When you feel the urge for a cigarette, do something else instead:
● Try going outside and breathing some fresh air.
● Take the dog for a walk.
● Do some exercises.
● Drink a glass of water.
● Clean your teeth.
● Chew some sugar-free gum, or a piece of carrot.
Congratulate yourself each time you manage to refuse a cigarette and each day you manage without a cigarette.

Work out how much smoking costs you financially as well as the costs to your health. Many people spend about £500 each year for 20 to 30 years – that is about £15,000 in total. Put all the money you would have spent on cigarettes in a jar and save up for something special such as a holiday.

Tell all your friends and family that you are giving up and ask for their help and support. If they smoke, ask them to try giving up with you – you can help each other – or ask them not to smoke in front of you or in the same room.

Keep a diary for a week and note down when you smoke and where. Try to avoid these situations for a while, until you have broken the habit.

If you have given up while in hospital, do everything you can to avoid starting again.

If you worry about putting on weight – don't! Most people gain only about 1–1.5kg/ 2–3lb when they stop smoking. It is less harmful to your health to gain a kilo or so in weight than to carry on smoking, and you can lose the excess weight once you have given up.

Do not fool yourself into cutting down to just one or two cigarettes a day or changing to a pipe or cigars. When you are under stress, you will find yourself back at your normal level of smoking.

When you have stopped, do not start again. Never smoke even the odd cigarette, otherwise you will soon find yourself falling back into the old routine.

Where to get help

Ask your doctor or practice nurse for help. They may run 'giving up smoking' groups. Ask them too for advice on nicotine patches, nasal spray or chewing gum. For information and support, phone Quitline on 0171 487 3000. Further information on the effects of smoking are available from ASH at the address on page 79.

Weight

About half the adults in Britain are overweight and this number is increasing. Are you one of these people? Find out by looking at the chart on page 27. Look at your weight on the vertical scale and your height on the horizontal scale and then look at where they cross over. You can then see whether you are a healthy weight.

Maintaining a healthy weight reduces your risk of heart disease, and you will also feel fitter and healthier. Your joints will work better as you get older too.

Going on a crash diet does not usually help in the long term. You may find it difficult to keep up, and many people end up putting more weight back on than they lost in the first place. You need to make changes to your diet and lifestyle which you can maintain long term. Aim for slow steady weight loss – about 0.5kg/1lb per week – rather than crash dieting.

Some ideas to help you to lose weight

- Try to have three meals each day. This will help you to stop snacking on high-calorie

Smoking, body weight and stress

snacks throughout the day. If you do not feel hungry at one of the mealtimes, still eat something; do not skip meals.

- Eat more slowly, chew each mouthful of food and put your cutlery down between each mouthful.
- Never shop for food on an empty stomach. Write a list of what you need and keep to it.
- Serve your food on smaller plates: then it will not look as if you are depriving yourself.
- Avoid buying fatty and high-calorie foods – do not tempt yourself.
- Keep a diary of what you eat and when (see below). Many people eat when they are upset, stressed or bored – hunger is usually at the bottom of the list. Why do you eat? When you have identified situations in which you end up eating between meals, try to avoid them.

- Get the support of your friends and family. Ask them not to offer you things to eat. Losing weight with a friend or partner may be easier.
- Increase your level of exercise: try to do some on most days. Choose a form that you enjoy – walking, swimming or cycling perhaps. Why not get family and friends to join in? Exercise will increase your metabolic rate, will help you to lose weight, and can be fun and enjoyable too. See pages 28–33 for more information, including details of a warm-up routine that is advised prior to any exercise session.

Other suggestions for improving your fitness

- Get off the bus one stop early.
- If you have a dog, take it for a walk. The dog will be happier and fitter too!

Food diary		
DAY	MONDAY	
Time	**Food**	**Reason for eating**
8 am	CORNFLAKES, TOAST & JAM	HUNGRY
9.30 am	CRISPS	FELT STRESSED
11 am	CHOCOLATE BAR	BORED

- Always use the stairs rather than the lift or escalator.
- Walk to the local shops or when going a short distance rather than taking the car or bus.
- Get your family or friends to join in and go for a walk or swim together.

Stress

What is stress? One dictionary definition is: mental, emotional, or physical strain or tension. Stress in moderation is actually part of normal life and keeps us motivated. Some people call this 'arousal'. If we had no stress, it would be difficult to keep going, but too much stress, especially if it is sustained over a long peroid, can be harmful.

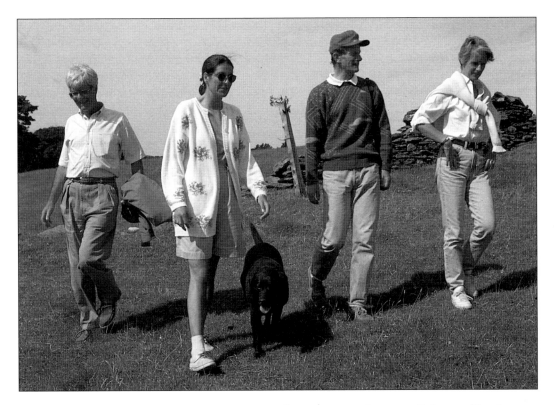

If you have a dog, take it for a good brisk walk and get some exercise yourself. Better still, take family and friends too.

Smoking, body weight and stress

If we cannot avoid stress, we have to learn to manage and cope with it. Excess stress is often thought of as the pressures on us which are beyond what we feel is tolerable, beyond our ability to cope.

Living with a heart condition is stressful; it is helpful, therefore, to learn more about stress and how to relax.

What happens when we experience stress?

When we meet a stressful situation, the hormones adrenaline and noradrenaline are secreted into the bloodstream. These cause the heart rate to be increased; raise the blood pressure; increase the blood flow to the muscles; reduce the blood flow to the gut and skin; cause the bronchi (tubes leading from the windpipe into the lungs) to expand, allowing more air to enter the lungs; and dilate the pupils. Adrenaline also causes glucose and fat to be released, ready to supply energy for the muscles. These changes are accompanied by increased alertness, leaving us ready to respond to further stimuli.

These stress responses helped us to survive when we lived in more primitive conditions where dangerous animals roamed, and would have prepared us to react either by running away from the danger or by fighting and tackling it. This is known as the 'fight or flight' mechanism. Nowadays these responses are not often required. It is usually inappropriate to run away from or physically fight whatever is causing the stress – for example, a long queue at the supermarket, another traffic jam, an interview or sheer frustration at work. This means that the body is preparing itself for actions which do not occur.

What causes stress?

Life events have been listed by psychologists in order of their impact on stress levels. Death of a spouse is thought to generate most stress and is at the top of the list, followed by divorce or separation, going to prison, death of a close family member, illness, marriage and loss of a job. Even a holiday is stress-provoking.

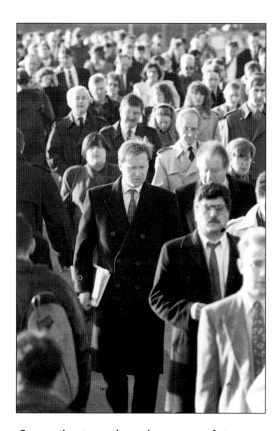

Commuting to work can be a cause of stress.

Some effects of stress

Stress affects different people in different ways. Some people cope better than others. Stress can result in many physical symptoms affecting different parts of the body and also mental symptoms. Some of these are listed below.

Poor sleep

Restlessness

Anxiety

Frustration

Exhaustion

Irritability

Undereating or overeating

Loss of self-esteem

Palpitations

Chest pain

Diarrhoea or upset stomach

Headaches

Giddiness

What is relaxation?

Deep relaxation is a way of letting go of stress and tension. Learning how to relax will help you to recover from your heart attack. Relaxation will help you to

● reduce stress and tension;

● cope with problems;

● lower your blood pressure;

● help you to sleep;

● help you to work more effectively;

● reduce angina.

Learning to relax takes time and practice. You need to practise every day for at least 20 minutes. At first you will find that your mind begins to wander. Do not be impatient – you cannot force yourself to relax.

How to relax

The first thing you need to do is to look at how you live. Get a pen and paper and write down the things in your life which cause you to become stressed. You can then try to think of ways in which you may be able to change some of these to make them less stressful, or even avoid stressful situations altogether. There will be some things that you cannot change, but if you can manage to make the list shorter you will have reduced your stress.

You can learn ways to cope with stressful events, simple exercises which you can carry out at any time. Write another list of things which you enjoy doing – hobbies, interests, sports, perhaps an evening class. Look in your local library for details of these, and try to think of ways in which you can increase the amount of time you spend on them.

Often if you are under stress you do not make time to do things that you enjoy. Set some time aside for yourself each day and spend it doing something that you enjoy. Perhaps you can set aside a longer period of time at the weekend. Let everyone know that this is your time for yourself and do not give in to pressure to spend this precious time doing something that you do not want to do. Spending more time doing something that you enjoy and less time on activities which cause you to be stressed will help you to feel more relaxed. You will also find that work will be put into better perspective, and you will go to work with a clearer and less tense mind.

Smoking, body weight and stress

Relaxation techniques

You probably have some way in which you unwind, such as having a warm bath, listening to music or watching television, but there are also specific relaxation techniques which you can learn.

Deep breathing

Find a comfortable chair to sit in or lie down on a bed or on the floor, making sure that you are comfortable and warm enough before you begin.

Place one hand on your chest and another on your stomach. Breathe in slowly through your nose and, when you feel that your lungs are full of air, hold your breath for a few seconds, then let the breath out slowly through your mouth; do not force this. Repeat several times. Notice which of your hands is moving up and down. The hand on your chest should not be moving, but the hand on your stomach should. Try to breathe so that your stomach moves in and out.

While you are doing this you may want to try closing your eyes and imagining you are lying on a beach on the warm sand listening to the waves lapping gently on the shore, with the warm sun shining on your body. Or in the countryside, lying on soft green grass by a small stream. Or imagine that you are in your favourite place, let your imagination take over and enjoy the relaxing experience.

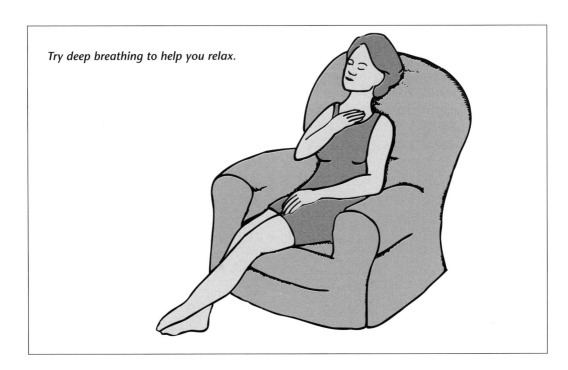

Try deep breathing to help you relax.

Progressive relaxation

This technique works by tensing and relaxing each group of muscles in your body in sequence. As you tense the muscles you can feel what you are trying to work against. You can carry out this exercise anywhere, and it takes between five and ten minutes to complete. Practise the technique at least once a day to gain full benefit. Do not worry if your mind begins to wander during the exercise; just refocus on the next group of muscles and carry on.

Again you need to start by finding a comfortable warm place to sit or lie. Close your eyes. Begin by focusing on your feet: try to tense all the muscles in your feet, hold on to the feeling of tension for a few seconds, then relax the muscles completely. When the muscles are relaxed, they will feel heavy. Repeat the exercise on the next group of muscles, those of the calf and thigh, then the buttocks, the stomach muscles, chest, hands and arms, shoulders and neck and finally the muscles of the face. When you have finished, you could do some deep-breathing exercises: as you breath out, imagine the stress and tension leaving your body.

Other ways to relax

You can buy tapes which talk you through relaxation techniques that some people find very useful. You may like to lie down and listen to some of your favourite music, and perhaps get one of your family or friends gently to massage your shoulders and neck. Some people find yoga or t'ai chi relaxing. Sometimes just going for a walk or swim helps; it gives you time away from the pressures to think and clear your mind.

At times throughout the day check the state of your muscles. Are they tense? If they are, try to relax them as described above.

Think positive

Many people find that they have negative thoughts after a heart attack or heart surgery, and these can be a source of stress. Thinking positive thoughts can help to overcome the problem.
- Most people make a full recovery after a heart attack.
- There are things that you can do to help your recovery.
- It is natural to tire more easily after a heart attack or heart surgery.
- The heart has amazing powers of recovery and can compensate for the damage.
- It is important to exercise and relax.
- Many people become fitter after a heart attack than they have been for years.
- When you are exercising, it is good to get *slightly* out of breath.

Smoking, body weight and stress

Sex after a heart attack

Many people are worried about when it will be safe to begin to have sex again. Sex is no different from any other form of exercise. If you are with your usual sexual partner in your own home, it puts as much strain on the heart as climbing two flights of stairs. Many people are afraid that sex will cause another heart attack, but this is actually very unlikely to happen. In cases where it has happened it is usually not with the person's usual partner and has occurred in a hotel room, after a heavy meal and a lot of alcohol.

Sex can help you to recover from your heart attack. If you become too breathless or begin to get chest pain, slow down or rest for a few minutes as you would with any form of exercise.

Your partner may be afraid that sex will lead to another heart attack, so may not seem very interested. If you think that this is happening, talk to each other about your worries and feelings. If this does not help, speak to your doctor together.

You may feel too tired. As you become fitter and take more exercise you will gradually find that you have more energy and your interest in sex will return. Stress can also reduce your desire for sex, so try to tackle your stress (see page 71).

If you find that you are having new problems, such as getting an erection, do not worry: the problem may go when you are feeling fitter and are more recovered. If you think it may be due to a side effect from a drug, do not stop taking the drug, but do talk to your doctor about it as there may be another drug which you can try.

If things do not improve, ask your doctor to refer you to someone who may be able to help, such as a clinical psychologist or a sexual counselling service. Do not suffer in silence.

How can family and friends help in the recovery process?

Family and/or friends often play an important role in recovery from heart attacks and heart surgery. They can provide physical and emotional support during the recovery process.

When you arrive home from hospital, you may be unable to carry out strenuous house-work, carry heavy shopping or drive for a while. Family and friends can often help until you are well enough to take over again. Although you may find it frustrating not being able to do what you used to, many families and friends like to help out in practical ways. But do not let them do everything; it is essential for your recovery that you do not retire to bed or to the nearest chair and let them wait on you hand and foot. You will be able to do some light housework and take some gentle exercise. You should have been given information before you were discharged from hospital on what to do. Gradually increase the things that you do.

Self-help groups

Self-help groups may help you to recover. You will meet other people who have been through the same experience, talking to them may help you and you will realize that you are not alone.

In time you yourself may be able to help others. Contact the British Heart Foundation (see page 79) for the addresses of groups near you.

Medical words explained

When you are reading about heart disease or talking to medical staff, they may use words which you do not understand. Here is an explanation of some of the words you may come across.

Aerobic exercise Exercise which causes the body to use more oxygen – for instance, brisk walking, swimming, jogging and cycling.

Angina Temporary attack of chest pain which may also extend to the shoulder or arm. The muscle of the heart becomes short of oxygen, which leads to pain. The pain may begin after exercise or stress, but can also occur at rest in some people.

Angiography A way of looking at the coronary arteries by passing a tube into the heart, injecting a liquid and taking X-ray pictures.

Angioplasty The coronary artery is widened by passing a balloon into the narrowed artery and inflating it.

Atheroma Fatty deposits in the walls of the blood vessels. The deposits cause the blood vessels to become narrower and weaken their walls, resulting in cracks inside the blood vessels on which clots can form.

Atherosclerosis This usually occurs at the same time as atheroma. The walls of the arteries become more rigid and less stretchy. It is another word for hardening of the arteries.

Blood pressure The pressure caused by the blood pressing on the blood vessel walls. It is measured with an instrument called a sphygmomanometer. A high blood pressure increases your chances of having a heart attack or stroke.

Cholesterol A fatty substance which is essential for life. It is used by the body to make cell walls, hormones, vitamin D and the bile salts which allow the body to digest fat. The body makes most of its own cholesterol in the liver. It is then moved around the body in the blood.

Corneal arcus A white ring around the outside of the coloured part of the eye. This can occur in older people for other reasons, but in younger adults can be one of the signs of familial hypercholesterolaemia (FH).

Smoking, body weight and stress

Coronary arteries The blood vessels which supply the heart with blood, carrying oxygen and food. These arteries can become narrowed or blocked, resulting in angina or heart attacks.

Electrocardiogram (ECG) This test measures the electrical activity of the heart. It helps doctors to see whether the heart is beating properly. It can also tell the doctor whether you have had a heart attack.

Familial hypercholesterolaemia (FH) Inherited high cholesterol. People with FH are at high risk of coronary heart disease at a young age. When blood triglyceride is raised as well as cholesterol, the condition is called familial combined hyperlipidaemia (FCH).

Fibrinogen A protein which circulates in the blood and can be converted to fibrin to form a blood clot.

HDL cholesterol HDL stands for high-density lipoprotein. HDL is known as 'good' cholesterol as it may help to clear excess cholesterol from the blood.

Hyperlipidaemia Too much of one or more of the fatty substances, cholesterol or triglyceride, in the blood.

Hypertension This is the medical term for high blood pressure.

LDL cholesterol LDL stands for low-density lipoprotein. This is known as 'bad' cholesterol. LDL cholesterol is the cholesterol which is deposited in the lining of the blood vessels.

Lipid Another name for fat. Fats are important as each cell in the body contains fats. Fats are also an important source of energy.

Lipoprotein$_{(a)}$, Lp$_{(a)}$ Low-density lipoprotein (LDL) can have an extra protein called apoprotein$_{(a)}$ attached to it. The whole complex is known as Lp$_{(a)}$. The extra (a) portion may stick to clots and interfere with their breakdown. High levels of Lp$_{(a)}$ in blood, as found in some patients with familial hypercholesterolaemia, may need extra attention.

Myocardial infarction (MI) Another name for a heart attack.

Triglyceride The name for fat as it is found in most animal and vegetable fats. It is the main form in which fat is stored in the body.

Xanthelasmata Pronounced 'zan-thel-as-mat-a', this describes deposits of cholesterol, usually yellow in colour, in the loose skin around the eye or eyelid.

Xanthoma Pronounced 'zan-thom-a'. It describes the condition in which cholesterol is deposited at the knuckles and tendons of the hands and elbows causing lumps to form. Cholesterol can also be deposited at the Achilles tendon at the back of each ankle, making it become thicker.

Unit conversion

Cholesterol: mmol/l x 38.6 = mg/dl
Triglycerides: mmol/l x 88.5 = mg/dl

Useful addresses

Family Heart Association
This organization provides information on coronary heart disease and its management by diet, lifestyle and drugs. Please write to the address below, enclosing an SAE.

Family Heart Association
7 High Street
Kidlington
Oxford OX5 2DH
Tel: 01865 370292

Alcohol Concern
275 Gray's Inn Road
London WC1X 8FQ
Tel: 0171 833 3471

Alcoholics Anonymous (AA)
PO Box 1
Stonebow House
Stonebow
York YO1 2NJ
Tel: 01904 644026

ASH (Action on Smoking and Health)
109 Gloucester Place
London W1H 3PH
Tel: 0171 935 3519

British Heart Foundation
14 Fitzhardinge Street
London W1H 3DA
Tel: 0171 935 0185

British Red Cross National Headquarters
9 Grovenor Crescent
London SW1X 7EJ
Tel: 0171 235 5454

Coronary Prevention Group
Plantation House
31–35 Fenchurch Street
London EC3M 3NN
Tel: 0171 626 4844

The Fish Foundation
PO Box 24
Tiverton
Devon EX16 4PQ
Tel: 01884 257 547

Health Education Authority
Hamilton House
Mabledon Place
London WC1H 9TX
Tel: 0171 383 3833

Meat and Livestock Commission
PO Box 44
Winterhill House
Snowdon Drive
Milton Keynes MK6 1AX
Tel: 01908 677577

National Dairy Council
John Princes Street
London W1M OAD
Tel: 0171 499 7822

National Drinkline National Alcohol Helpline
London only
Tel: 0171 332 0202
All UK (calls charged at local rate)
Tel: 0345 320202
Dial and Listen Service
Tel: Freecall 0500 801 802

Smokers' Helpline

England
Quitline
102 Gloucester Place
London W1H 3DA
Tel: 0171 487 3000

Scotland
Tel: 0800 848484

Northern Ireland
01232 663281

Wales
01222 641888

The Stroke Association
CHSA House
Whitecross Street
London EC1Y 8JJ
Tel: 0171 490 7999
Provides information on stroke and blood pressure

The St John Ambulance National Headquarters
1 Grovenor Crescent
London SW1X SEF
Tel: 0171 235 5231

Eire

Irish Heart Foundation
4 Clyde Road
Ballsbridge
Dublin 4

Northern Ireland

Northern Ireland Chest, Heart and Stroke Association
21 Dublin Road
Belfast BT2 7FJ

Australia

National Heart Foundation of Australia
National Office
PO Box 2
Woden
A.C.T. 2606

Canada

Canadian Association for Familial Hypercholesterolaemia
PO Box 846
Place du Parc
Montreal (QC)
H2W 2P5

USA

American Heart Association
National Center
7320 Greenville Avenue
Dallas
Texas 75231

The Center for the Prevention of Heart Disease
Park Center Medical Building
1200 North Tustin Avenue
Suite 100
Santa Ana
California 92705

National Cholesterol Education Program
National Heart, Lung and Blood Institute
National Institutes of Health
C–200
Bethesda
Maryland 20892

Index

W A R D   L O C K

FAMILY HEALTH GUIDE

LIVING WITH A
HEART CONDITION

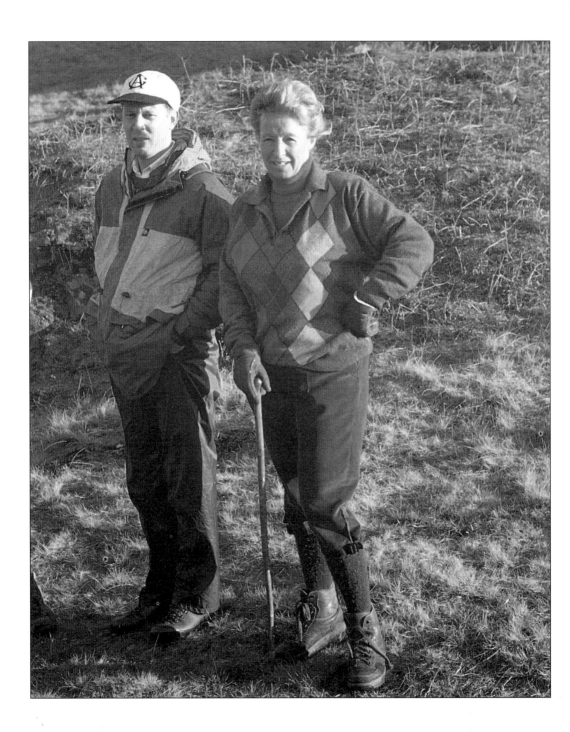

Lumen — Smooth muscle cells and wall

Reducing your cholesterol

Age (years)	Reduction in risk of heart attack (%)
40	50
50	40
60	30
70	20

This table shows the reduction in risk of having a heart attack by a 10% reduction in total blood cholesterol at different ages.
Source: British Medical Journal, 1994.

Low-density lipoprotein (LDL)
Carries cholesterol from the liver, where it is made, around the body to the tissues where it is used.
High-density lipoprotein (HDL)
Carries surplus cholesterol not used by the tissues back to the liver for disposal.
Triglyceride (TG)
Ordinary fat used as a 'fuel'. It is transported in lipoproteins, especially in VLDLs and chylomicrons.

Very low-density lipoprotein (VLDL)
Transports triglycerides from where they are made around the body to the tissues where they are used.
Chylomicrons
Especially rich in triglycerides. They transport dietary fat absorbed in the intestines to the liver for processing and to fat tissues for storage.